SECOND (GENERAL) EDITION
(Updated January 2022)

ARTIFICIAL INTELLIGENCE IN HEALTHCARE

PARAG MAHAJAN, MD

MedMantra, LLC
New Mexico

Second Edition of "ARTIFICIAL INTELLIGENCE IN HEALTHCARE " by
Parag Mahajan, MD

MedMantra, LLC

1330 San Pedro Drive NE STE 205A, Albuquerque, NM 87110

MedMantra.com

ISBN: 978-93-5351-683-3 (Paperback)

ISBN: 978-93-5351-845-5 (eBook)

Copyright © 2022 MedMantra, LLC

Register your copy:

First edition: July 2018 | Second edition: April 2019 | Third edition: February 2021

The 2nd edition was first updated and renamed as "General Edition" in April 2021 and further updated in January 2022

The 3rd edition was first updated and renamed as "Academic Edition" in April 2021 and further updated in January 2022

Register your copy of this book by following the instructions mentioned at MedMantra.com/aih

Registration entitles you to a completely free eBook of the next edition/update.

Speaker invitations and business consultation requests:

Contact the author by email (DrParag@MedMantra.com) for speaker invitations or business consultation requests.

DEDICATION

Nobody has been more important to me in the pursuit of writing this book than the members of my family. I would like to thank my parents, whose love and encouragement are with me in whatever I pursue. I would especially like to mention the forever cheerful attitude of my father, who maintained it even while recently being treated for stomach cancer. Most importantly, I wish to thank my loving and supportive wife, Anuradha, and my two wonderful daughters, Anoushka and Paavni, who provide unending inspiration. I would also like to thank my role models, Elon Musk and Stephen Hawking, who inspired me to delve into the quest of the unknown.

Artificial Intelligence (AI) in Healthcare - Professional Certification Courses - 100% Online

Learn at your own pace from the comfort of your home

Pioneered by MedMantra Academy

- **Level 1 (Basic) Course** (12 Modules) - **2-24 Weeks**
- **Level 2 (Executive) Course** (20 Modules) - **4-24 Weeks**
- **Level 3 (Expert) Course / Healthcare AI Application Programing Course** (10+ Projects & 3+ Tutorials) - **2-24 Weeks**
- **Courses starting from US$ 99**

ENROLL NOW!

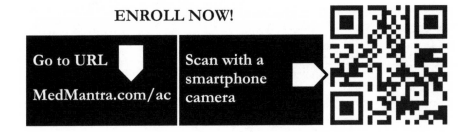

Go to URL	Scan with a smartphone camera
MedMantra.com/ac	

Claim Your Surprise Gift

Thank you for checking out my book. To show my appreciation, I've prepared a special gift for all my readers that will help you master all aspects of artificial intelligence in healthcare. The gift is in the form of regularly updated & free bonus articles, videos, training courses, and lots more...

Access it by visiting: MedMantra.com/aih

Check out the "Academic Edition 2022" of this book for comprehensive details on AI in Healthcare

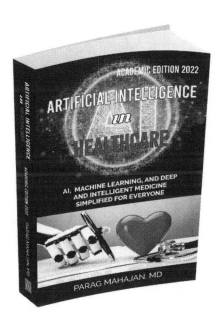

Features:

- The most authoritative text on the subject.

- Details on the implementation of AI in clinical practice.

- AI's role in medical research & education, health insurance, drug discovery, electronic health records, genomic & precision medicine, telehealth, healthcare robotics, COVID-19, & more.

- Detailed discussion on the ethics of AI in healthcare.

- Detailed & simplified explanation about machine learning & data science.

- Latest updates about the current applications & future of AI in healthcare & all major medical specialties.

- Further details here: **MedMantra.com/aih**

TABLE OF CONTENTS

"The question of whether a computer can think is no more interesting than the question of whether a submarine can swim."

- Edsger W. Dijkstra

SECTION 1
ARTIFICIAL INTELLIGENCE IN HEALTHCARE

CHAPTER ONE

ARTIFICIAL INTELLIGENCE VERSUS HUMAN INTELLIGENCE

Artificial intelligence is a broad term that encompasses any code, algorithm, or combined technology designed to mimic human intelligence or behavior. Various subdomains make up this entity we commonly refer to as AI. Every AI-based technology can be applied to a different aspect of human ability.

Think of artificial intelligence as the "man-made" form of all human processes. *In simple terms, AI is a machine, device, robot, or tool that is powered by software programmed to display the characteristic reasoning and thinking patterns of humans.* To date, these machines have achieved specific purposes by reacting to specific actions according to how they have been programmed—that is, the data sets that they have used as learning material.

Most of us use AI in our daily lives without even realizing it. The most prevalent way is its reach into social media for the development of marketing strategies that use AI-powered algorithms to evaluate consumer behavior. From browsing history to shopping history to movie choices, our internet actions give companies like *Netflix, Amazon,* and *Facebook* a detailed database for market analysis. Companies like *Ayzenberg*[1] developed proprietary intelligent algorithms that capture user-generated data to analyze and predict market trends. Years ago, *Boeing* introduced its AI-powered autopilot feature. Also, car manufacturer *Tesla*[2] stepped up its game by providing recent models with Autopilot features. Tesla's self-driving technology is based on an AI-backed system that detects a car's surroundings and navigates the car accordingly. Facial recognition software used at passport control in airport security, as well as virtual assistants like *Siri, Alexa,* and *Google Home,* use responsive AI technology to function.

The concept of AI seems to differ for everyone. Some people consider it to be the ultimate solution to all the problems that humankind faces. For others, its use is limited to specific sectors. For a data scientist, AI holds a whole different meaning. To them, AI is a means to an end—a tool meant to provide both social and monetary benefits by analyzing large datasets, too enormous for the human mind to compute. AI software can be programmed to detect complex patterns, which then lead to predictive actions that are most likely to bring about success.

Artificial intelligence is generally categorized into two parts: generalized and applied AI. The focus of applied AI is more on robotics, which constructs programs that enable these systems to perform tasks just as well as a human being could. Generalized AI, on the other hand, encompasses the development of machines that can mimic human intelligence, while analyzing data and predicting actionable outcomes. AI works through a programming sequence in which the program's central point is defined. It may be very easy to underestimate the potential of AI, due to the assumption that it is simply an advanced computer program following predetermined rules laid out by human programmers or coders. Historically, creating and applying software has followed the principles of an "if - then - else" function— that is, if a desired outcome is not achieved after the software works on the input data, corrections are made in the system until the desired outcome is achieved. This is often done through trial and error and may be extremely time-consuming.

Here is where the application of generalized AI was an absolute game changer! By introducing machine learning (ML) as a solution, we allow the *program* to learn from provided examples or practice data sets, and then *apply* this knowledge to new data sets in order to recognize patterns and provide probable outcomes … *exhibiting human intelligence.* It can continuously and automatically *correct and adjust* its calculations to produce the desired output. Deep learning (DL) is a subset of machine learning, which uses artificial neural networks to mimic human decision-making by imbibing large data sets in order to properly understand and analyze a concept, and then provide a meaningful outcome. These artificial neural networks use math and computer science principles to imitate the processes of densely interconnected brain cells, using neurons, or nodes that are built from code.

So, how does all this technology translate into real-world scenarios? Here is an example to make things clear. Imagine that you are the owner of an e-commerce business. You want to know what product a customer is likely to purchase at a given time. To accomplish this, you would need a *predictive modeler*, which will look at the buying history and choices of that particular customer to predict what the customer is more likely to buy. The theory revolves around understanding the complex behavior of buyers and accurately predicting the decisions they will make. This helps the manufacturers and providers plan their products purposefully while avoiding waste. At the same time, the customers can find more of what they want in the market, creating a win-win situation for both parties. The factors that the predictor uses can vary from case to case. Some factors that can influence the outcome include:

- Climate

- Factors related to demography, such as the marital status of the customer, as well as the customer's profession, education, and age

- Opinion of any partner and the resulting impact

- Alternate options available at the time

- Environmental factors

These are merely a few points and it is nearly impossible to compile a whole list of consumer behaviors. Considering the massive list of factors, it is clear that there would be innumerable possibilities. If we consider the probability of these factors affecting the choice of the buyer, estimating these permutations and combinations is too large and daunting a task for a single human being to accomplish with any degree of success. This is where AI and machine learning step in to save the day!

With a combination of the right hardware, smart software, and detailed data, an AI-based machine learning system can operate seamlessly to find a fool-proof equation that would integrate and analyze the data that it is fed. While generating one-time solutions is an incredible feat by itself, the beauty of an ML system is its ability to continuously improve its performance. The system memorizes all the possible suggestions or solutions it created with every analysis, retaining the applicable or sound solutions in memory while discarding those that do not seem appropriate. This is simple learning or programming of a higher order, which has the potential for massive, exciting applications in the future.

It is, however, important to keep in mind that, at present, an ML program still needs human assistance to operate optimally. It is our responsibility to keep a check on what kind of data, as well as how much data, is provided to it, as at the end of the day, statistics is a numbers game. An AI algorithm cannot figure out causation on its own, which is what separates it from absolute human cognition and intelligence. The system cannot be expected to determine things that are not introduced through the data input or reference points that human beings provide to the algorithm. The reference points are basically the permissible deviations in the equations entered. These are vital for learning, and ML and DL algorithms will fail to evolve in their absence.

AI in Practice: Man versus Machine

A voice robot can be used to illustrate the working of AI algorithms in practice. The interactive voice response, or IVR, used in the patients' service line in a busy hospital is utilized to make things clear. In this imaginary interaction between man and machine, AI is represented by the voice robot and Pt denotes a patient.

Pt: *I have a skin problem. I need to consult a dermatologist.*
AI: *I understand, ma'am. Is this an emergency or can you wait?*
Pt: *It's not an emergency, but I need the earliest available appointment.*
AI: *Okay, ma'am. Would you like an appointment with Dr. Richard or Dr. Lisa?*
Pt: *Dr. Richard, please.*
AI: *The earliest available appointment with Dr. Richard is this Wednesday, the 5th. Shall I book it for 6:30 pm?*
Pt: *Yes, please.*
AI: *Can you please share your name, mobile number, and insurance details?*
Pt: *"Supplies answers."*
AI: *Thank you for the details, Angela.*

While the interaction may seem simple on the surface, an extremely complex sequence of events made this conversation possible. When we speak, a speech signal is derived. The waves of amplitude are plotted by the computer programmed with ML capabilities. The audio signals are then used to distinguish *cepstral features*, which include:

- Amplitude

- Variation between sound waves

- Distance between two wave cycles

- Distance between the lowest trough and the highest wave

AI is responsible for converting these signals into a spoken English language that can be understood by all. How is this done? By feeding it with the speech signals, along with the related transcripts. This is similar to a situation in which a teacher writes the letter "C "on the blackboard and tells a student that this is, in fact, the letter "C". The student then memorizes the image and the relevant sounds or phonics associated with the letter, as well as the context in which they may be used. Similarly, when related texts along with the speech signals are provided to a machine learning algorithm, the AI can use continuous, complex, and abstract learning to:

1. Classify the patient's speech;

2. Match the speech signals to the transcript of the conversation, as well as to its own historical, stored text memory;

3. Provide a seamless, human-like interaction, in which it can understand the customer's words and reply accordingly.

Artificial intelligence versus Human intelligence – The Verdict

AI systems, both applied and generalized, can learn from historical data. An AI system then further defines the parameters by using the next level of pattern recognition, thus completing its job. The question is: Can you attain a higher level than this?

Taking the example of the interactive voice response software explained earlier, what happens if something out of the ordinary occurs, like the patient develops a sore throat? Would the system still be able to transform the speech into text? AI-based software cannot adjust to unpredicted scenarios without adequate training, while human beings, by nature, are known to evolve and adapt to new situations by logically processing changes in their environments. In comparison, a machine can learn only what it is taught. Thus, it can adapt to this change only if it is fed with new signals, new information, or new data sets that can then generate a revised, relevant, and accurate output.

At the moment, it is safe to say that while significant progress has been made to simulate human intelligence, AI has not been able to evolve to a degree such that it can completely replace human thought and intervention. After all, human beings made machines in the first place. This gives rise to the question: Where does AI technology fall short?

1. *Sensory information:*

    Human beings possess five synchronized senses, which are impossible to replicate in machines. For example, a self-driven car may make its way flawlessly through traffic, but it will never be able to appreciate the delicious aroma of freshly brewed coffee from the café it just passed.

2. *Creativity:*

    This is where humans excel! The varied languages, the nuances of regional dialects, the casual abbreviations, and the tone and expression of the spoken word can be completely lost on machine learning algorithms. Can you imagine soul-searching poetry written by a machine? Or a piece of art that strikes a chord with your emotions, painted by a robot? For the moment, the reins of creativity lie in the hands of humans, along with the personality that expresses it.

3. *Deductive reasoning:*

    While AI could arguably arrive at logical conclusions in perfectly synchronized events much faster and probably with greater accuracy than humans can, deductive reasoning often requires out-of-the-box thinking that is unattainable for even the most advanced software. After all, the greatest detective in the world had both a brilliant brain and an empathetic heart, which worked hand in hand to help him solve his mysteries! This is possible only because of flawed and imperfect human emotions and thoughts, which manage to disrupt the natural deduction of a perfectly logical data set—much to the chagrin of the AI software.

4. *Judgment:*

On the same note, the ability to judge complicated and intricate situations with clarity, as well as ethically and with moral responsibility, is purely a human ability. While machines can diagnose health conditions or calculate mathematical equations with a high degree of accuracy, discriminating between morally right and wrong decisions is way beyond their scope at the moment.

5. *Right brain thinking:*

According to scientists, the human brain uses its right side to empathize with others, giving rise to a gut feeling or intuition several years in the making. The mind can understand imminent threats and dangers. For instance, when we see someone drowning on TV, we can think about how he must have felt while losing his breath. This is what enables us to empathize with those facing problems, even if they are disconnected.

6. *Social behavior:*

Human beings are social animals and develop relationships and interact with each other in ways that sometimes defy logic. The currently available AI-powered machines are not social and, so, are unable to arrive at conclusions that humans may end up at.

As exciting as the innovations in AI technology are, the fact is, as humans, we are sentient beings that have evolved to survive by making our own energy, software, and hardware.

We are also armed with emotional energy that allows us to push the envelope, crossing the realms of reasoning. Our thinking ability enables us to unleash our creativity when we most need it. The human brain is capable of running many simulations without facing the danger of breaking down. To date, no machine can achieve this, as they are incapable of surviving without users and manufacturers.

The concept of man versus machine is merely a figment of imagination at this point, something restricted to movies. The ground reality, however, begs to differ!

CHAPTER TWO

A BRIEF INTRODUCTION TO AI
IN HEALTHCARE

Artificial intelligence (AI) is a young discipline [see Figure 2-1] that is here to bring a paradigm shift to healthcare. While it cannot replace doctors or healthcare workers in the foreseeable future, it is certainly poised to bring about a foundational shift in medical systems worldwide. With AI permeating every aspect of daily life, is it really a surprise that AI has found its way into the healthcare sector as well?

AI and Its Foray into Healthcare

While there are practical applications of AI in all human facets, the use of these tools in the field of healthcare shows remarkable potential for growth. Research has shown that the AI in healthcare market is expected to reach $120 billion by 2028, with an annual compounded growth rate of over 40%. It is also predicted to reduce annual healthcare costs by $150 billion by 2026.[3]

The adoption of AI-backed medical devices has only recently improved, with the United States Food and Drug Administration (FDA) approving the technology for patient use in 2017 and the Ministry of Food and Drug Safety in Korea approving it in 2018.[4]

The medical industry generates a tremendous amount of information every day [see Figure 2-2]. The use of technology to stratify and centralize this data to ensure easy accessibility has been the need of healthcare professionals for a very long time. The data available in the form of electronic health records (EHRs), X-rays, ECGs, and lab reports can be entered into algorithms for the training of AI models. AI can then develop its own "logic," which will empower medical personnel in an integrated system that translates useful information into functional tools. The ability of AI-enabled systems to work flawlessly in mimicking human cognition has dominated the rhetoric. The AI has helped healthcare in integrating statistical analysis, fast and accurate diagnosis, and the development of life-critical applications.[4]

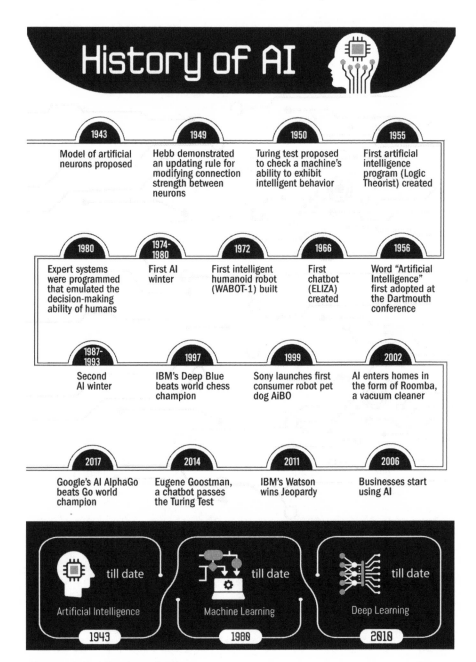

Figure 2-1. History of AI

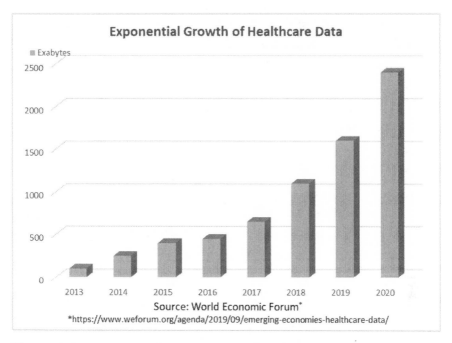

Figure 2-2. Exponential growth of healthcare data

Let us now understand the terms and acronyms commonly used with AI:

1. *Machine Learning* (ML) is a subdomain of AI involving the techniques and processes that help the machine to develop its own logic through self-learning. This knowledge can then be used to analyze patterns in large volumes of images, like making an image-based diagnosis in the fields of radiology and pathology. It can also be applied to discover anomalies in genomic structures, which can help diagnose congenital or gene-mediated diseases.

2. *Deep Learning* (DL) is a specific type of machine learning described as the modern revival of artificial neural networks (ANNs). ANNs are algorithms that mimic the biological structure of the brain. Deep learning can train AI algorithms to statistically analyze large amounts of data to accurately predict patient treatment results as well as provide personalized recommendations to patients regarding their treatment plans.

3. ***Robotics*** incorporates technological precision with an AI-enabled accurate diagnosis to enhance surgical procedures and can be used extensively in the medical device industry.

4. ***Natural Language Processing (NLP) and Voice Recognition*** can convert long-form, unstructured patient information commonly found in transcribed physician notes or electronic medical records into classified and formatted data that then becomes easy to analyze and interpret.

5. ***Predictive Modeling*** applies mathematical methods and tools to large data sets to forecast patient conditions or prognoses by using retrospective information for prospective action.

Bringing AI to the Patient

The dawn of the Internet of Things gave way to ***the Internet of Medical Things (IoMT)***, which brought a whole new dimension to the application of AI-enabled software directly into the patient's hands. Access to technology is no longer limited to healthcare providers or medical device and pharmaceutical companies. With wearable technology in the form of fitness bands, smartwatches, smart oximeters, and glucometers connected to smartphone applications and analytical software, patients and users have direct access to health information. They can analyze, interpret, and act on their own health data, approaching physicians for consultations earlier for interventions. This focus on preventive health has gained predominance in recent years, with tech giants like Apple, Google, Samsung, and IBM competing to commercialize services, applications, and devices that integrate AI tools to improve diagnostic and prognostic accuracy.

A recent study done by *Hannun and colleagues*[5] used a deep learning algorithm to analyze 91,232 single-lead ECGs. The AI was able to diagnose abnormal readings with ECG pattern recognition as well as trained cardiologists.

In 2017, Apple[6] and Samsung[7] applied deep learning algorithms to their smartwatches, which were able to detect atrial fibrillation through an inbuilt ECG monitor and heart rate readings. This received FDA approval and is widely used by consumers to date.

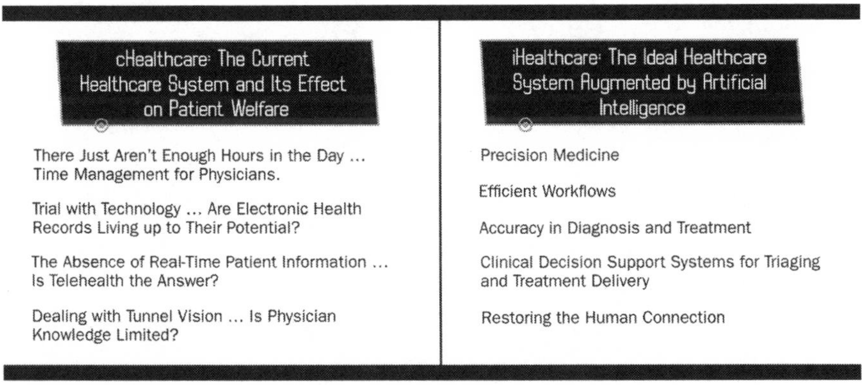

cHealthcare: The Current Healthcare System and Its Effect on Patient Welfare	iHealthcare: The Ideal Healthcare System Augmented by Artificial Intelligence
There Just Aren't Enough Hours in the Day ... Time Management for Physicians.	Precision Medicine
	Efficient Workflows
Trial with Technology ... Are Electronic Health Records Living up to Their Potential?	Accuracy in Diagnosis and Treatment
The Absence of Real-Time Patient Information ... Is Telehealth the Answer?	Clinical Decision Support Systems for Triaging and Treatment Delivery
Dealing with Tunnel Vision ... Is Physician Knowledge Limited?	Restoring the Human Connection

Figure 2-3. cHealthcare and iHealthcare

cHealthcare: The Current Healthcare System and Its Effect on Patient Welfare

While the rapid application of AI principles to healthcare is undoubtedly exciting, with its boundless potential to improve global health and wellness efforts, it is important to understand WHY its application was required and what factors in the current system inspired its widespread adoption. It is human nature to learn and evolve from situations that are detrimental to the longevity and quality of life, so it is but natural to infer that there were gaps in the existing healthcare facilities that facilitated the innovation required for AI-based technology. If we consider the current healthcare system (referred to *as cHealthcare*, from this point) with an objective eye, its flaws are apparent.

1. *There Just Aren't Enough Hours in the Day ... Time Management for Physicians.*

When it comes to creating a relationship between doctor and patient, a series of issues come into play. One of the main things that isn't always considered is the fact that doctors must spend adequate time with patients to make sure they understand what the patient is going through. Unfortunately, there is a serious dearth of this valuable time, and physician visits always seem rushed and haphazard. Research has demonstrated that patient satisfaction is directly dependent on the quality of communication with healthcare providers.

13

Ludmerer noted, "For over a century, the goal of medical education has been to produce thinking physicians, scientifically competent, who are sensitive to the emotional as well as the medical condition of the patient".[8]

Ninety-three percent of all human communication is based on body language, while only 7% is dependent on the exchange of words. Physicians struggling with increased workloads will find themselves running out of time and rushing through patient interactions. These distracted visits are noted by patients, who tend to lose trust in their providers as a result.[9,10]

Contrary to popular belief, this overload is rarely due to an increase in patient load. However, systems worldwide are so dependent on recording and documentation of patient interactions that most physicians and other medical experts are busy trying to keep up with the data that is constantly being provided to them. There is a continual need to fill in patient notes, transcribe patient information, and input patient data into paper files or electronic systems, which may be handled by scribes or physician assistants in some cases, but which is still dependent largely on skilled manual labor. This situation is similar in both outpatient clinics and inpatient care.

A study in 2018, conducted in an intensive care unit of a hospital, used a sensor network to analyze how long healthcare workers spent in direct patient contact. The study aimed to be more accurate than traditional surveys, which were subject to participants' memories or human observers, which themselves were prone to observational bias. The results of the study demonstrated that physicians spent 14.7% of their shift time in patient rooms or at bedsides, while they spent 40% of their time in the physician workroom, tied to their desks, busy with electronic medical record review and documentation. This limited interaction with patients further fuels patient dissatisfaction and distrust, as patients perceive it as indicative of substandard care delivery.[11]

There was also a concern regarding the lack of real-time information about patients, apart from time spent at the clinic. The rationale was that patients are not diagnosed based on data from their daily lives. With limited face-to-face interactions during physical consultations, the doctors can offer insight only into obvious findings without a holistic view of the patient's health status.

2. *The Absence of Real-Time Patient Information ... Is Telehealth the Answer?*

Before the COVID-19 pandemic in 2020, doctors generally did not have time to follow up with patient information after patient visits, considering their ongoing workload. While an accurate diagnosis is dependent on the patient's ability to recall their symptoms or experiences with medication for their next in-person visit with their doctor, it is natural for this information to be unreliable or incomplete. 2020 provided a turning point for this physician-patient interaction with the introduction of remote patient monitoring devices linked to smartphone applications that could easily be shared with one's healthcare provider. This was a demonstration of necessity being the mother of invention, as social distancing mandates pushed for greater adoption of telehealth facilities, with more patients opting for wearable digital health technology to monitor and evaluate their health matrices. This included smartwatches, fitness bands, blood pressure and heart rate monitors, pulse oximeters, and glucometers, which captured real-time patient information for rapid analysis. Many of these applications were backed by AI software, resulting in rapid, real-time physiological monitoring and greater compliance. The constant monitoring and generation of large data volumes proved to be another hurdle to conquer ... because now that we had a way to automatically capture this data, how would we analyze it and then act on it?[12]

3. *Trial with Technology ... Are Electronic Health Records Living up to Their Potential?*

The introduction of electronic health records (EHRs) undoubtedly has created an advantage over paper-based systems that were prone to errors and lapses in communication and continuity of care. With enhanced patient data security and the ease with which reports and patient information can be transferred from one physician to another, patients are protected from unnecessary testing, duplication of diagnostic testing, and medication errors. With better electronic medical records, it will also be easier to correlate genomic data with phenotypic data for patients.

However, the accuracy of this data is largely dependent on physicians, who enter the data themselves through charting, round notes, or handoff notes. It seems that once again, a solution to one problem opened Pandora's box and let loose another set of issues to overcome. There is a difference between being active and being productive. Electronic health records have been linked to cognitive overload and user burnout. According to the National Physician Burnout and Suicide Report 2020, which evaluated 15,000 physicians in over 29 specialties, 42% of participants reported being burnt out, while 55% of the respondents cited bureaucratic tasks like data entry, charting, and administrative work as the primary cause for burnout.

A large amount of data present in electronic medical records must be properly analyzed and interpreted for it to be used to its full potential. The application of artificial intelligence algorithms is necessary to wade through the overwhelming data sets and arrive at actionable conclusions to improve care delivery. Otherwise, it is very easy to lose sight of the objective and drown in data.

Dr. Erica Shenoy, MD, PhD, Associate Chief of the Infection Control Unit at Massachusetts General Hospital, Boston, USA, noted, "AI tools can live up to the expectation for infection control and antibiotic resistance. If they don't, then that's really a failure on all of our parts. For the hospitals sitting on mountains of EHR data and not using them to the fullest potential, to industry that's not creating smarter, faster clinical trial design, and for EHRs that are creating this data not to use them ... that would be a failure".[13]

4. *Dealing with Tunnel Vision ... Is Physician Knowledge Limited?*

Physicians have been known to concentrate on the patient at hand, limited by the knowledge they have already attained, simply because they may not have the time to research or compare their patient status with those in large databases, with the unlimited case studies or references available in the medical literature. The research takes too long, and the interpretation of study findings is often inconclusive and may not apply to their patient demographics, which in turn makes them fall back on comfortable and repetitive models of diagnosis and treatment. This raises a pertinent question about the practical utilization of medical studies that are published.

Despite the obvious value of medical literature, it is extremely challenging for physicians to keep up with the latest advances in their fields. A report in the Journal of the American Medical Library Association found that over 7,000 articles are published monthly in primary care journals alone.[14]

Medical practice has a "TL;DR (Too Long; Didn't Read)" problem. Most physicians may not have the time to keep themselves updated with the latest advancements in their specialties. In recognition of this problem, a research project used artificial intelligence programs to comb through vast medical literature databases to derive results for focused themed research. The AI scored 49 out of 60 points, outperforming the human researchers, who scored 46 points using the same matrices for research accuracy. This shows the potential that AI has to analyze and filter required information to facilitate improved medical education.[15]

The varied factors responsible for the lacunae in *eHealthcare* are also the factors that lead to ***misdiagnosis***, which further fragments an already-fragile doctor-patient relationship.

When patients are diagnosed with the wrong illness and offered treatments that are not suitable to their needs, the result will generally be worsened patient care delivery, increased mortality and morbidity rates associated with inflated medical malpractice premiums, and the risk of legal repercussions for healthcare providers.

Reports on the economics of medical errors have revealed that medical errors cost the United States $19.5 billion per annum. In addition, the annual costs of "defensive medicine," which constitutes unnecessary investigations ordered solely to protect physicians from malpractice suits, are valued at $45-60 billion US per annum. This shines a light on the wastage of resources, time, and energy on treatment modalities that do not have a robust evidence base or clinical decision support.[16,17]

With all that can potentially go wrong in cHealthcare, does artificial intelligence have what it takes to improve the current scenario and bring much-needed reforms and support to clinical care?

iHealthcare: The Ideal Healthcare System Augmented by Artificial Intelligence

While AI doesn't aim to replace human doctors in the current healthcare system, it does have a goal to make the system more effective.

What was considered science fiction is now within our grasp. This thought brings excitement and apprehension in equal parts to the minds of healthcare providers worldwide. An imagined utopia—a healthcare system powered by AI-enabled tools and software—seems to be right around the corner. The extent to which algorithms and machine learning will penetrate the medical industry remains to be seen. If we consider this AI-driven healthcare industry (referred to as *iHealthcare* from this point), we can evaluate how making use of both human effort and advanced technology can bring us closer to efficiency and accuracy in the field of medicine.

1. *Precision Medicine*

Precision medicine has gained traction since the introduction of AI in healthcare, as it shows the immense possibilities in customizing care delivery or delivering solutions based on an individual patient's genetics, lifestyle, location, and environmental factors. This is opposed to the one-size-fits-all approach that traditional medicine delivers. It spans the treatment journey from diagnosis to disease detection, prognosis, and management. By taking advantage of AI algorithms, genomic and proteomic profiles of patient subgroups can be analyzed to predict risk factors for cardiovascular disease and cancer as well as prognostic factors for neurodegenerative conditions.

In the last few years, the digitization of medical records added large amounts of patient data with initiatives from the NIH (USA) called the EMERGE network and the "All of Us" program, databases from the Canadian Institutes of Health Research, and the National Health Service, UK. The application of AI algorithms to these data sets can help to derive genotype-phenotype relationships for specific genetic diseases, with the ability to deliver holistic care to patients. AI algorithms aided in the mapping of the human genome, which, along with the addition of MRI images, helped to establish the Allen Developmental Brain Atlas in 2011 and the Human Cell Atlas in 2017. This can lead to personalized treatments with FDA-approved targeted gene therapy.[18] The Tempus group[19] has developed its AI software to provide a large library of clinical and molecular data that enables doctors to make real-time decisions for data-driven, personalized therapeutics.

2. *Efficient Workflows*

AI in healthcare will build on systems with automation and robotics to deliver better care outcomes through a lean management strategy that reduces wastage of resources for healthcare providers while delivering value-based care to patients. The **McKinsey Group** has estimated that AI will help in the automation of 15% of current working hours in the healthcare industry.[20]

US-based company **Olive**[21] has a machine learning algorithm that automates repetitive tasks in healthcare management, thereby freeing physicians and administrators to work on more pressing issues. The platform can automate insurance checks and claims and seamlessly integrates with a healthcare network to track down deficiencies and highlight areas for improvement. **CloudMedX**[22] uses deep learning to generate analysis that showcases areas of improvement in the patient's journey through the healthcare system. Its coding analyzer was used with existing coding and billing software to efficiently manage, analyze, and communicate structured and unstructured data to improve patient care.

3. *Accuracy in Diagnosis and Treatment*

Machine and deep learning algorithms are experts at pattern recognition and image analysis, which greatly improves the accuracy of radiological and pathological diagnoses.

Digital pathology platforms like **Proscia**[23] improve the speed and accuracy of cancer diagnostics, while **Zebra Medical Vision**[24] arms radiologists with an AI-powered assistant that analyzes and filters routine scans from those with positive clinical findings to help lighten the workload for practitioners.

4. *Clinical Decision Support Systems for Triaging and Treatment Delivery*

Clinical decision support tools have existed for years but are attracting attention now due to the application of AI algorithms to existing electronic data through health records or imaging reports.

A study conducted by **Pickhardt and colleagues**[25] used body composition markers from abdominal CT scans to develop a deep learning algorithm focused on imaging features, as compared to clinical parameters like Framingham Risk Scores and Body Mass Index (BMI), to predict major cardiovascular disease as well as survival rates for adult patient populations. The algorithm outperformed established clinical indicators.

5. *Restoring the Human Connection*

AI-enabled systems have the potential to reduce the cognitive load that overwhelms physicians and leads to increased incidents of burnout. The World Health Organization (WHO) states, "Although the global economy could create 40 million new health-sector jobs by 2030, there is still a projected shortfall of 9.9 million physicians, nurses and midwives globally over the same period." The automation of repetitive, time-consuming processes through AI-enabled systems also addresses the issue of shortage in manpower while aiding in the provision of care services to underserved or developing areas.[26] It is ironic that many believe the application of AI will, or the adoption of technology in diagnosis and treatment may cause, further detachment between physicians and patients by establishing additional barriers. However, it may result in just the opposite effect because it has the potential to free physicians from routine and mundane tasks so that they can provide empathy and re-establish a human connection in the doctor-patient dynamic—a skill that cannot be replaced even with the most advanced AI. In other words, AI will allow doctors to be more … human.

Potential Liabilities with the Application of AI in Healthcare

As with most things in life, all that glitters is not gold. While AI is often touted as a concept that will revolutionize medicine and care delivery, evaluating it with a critical eye is bound to reveal inconsistencies and lacunae in its development and implementation that may make us accept the claims of its potential with a pinch of salt.

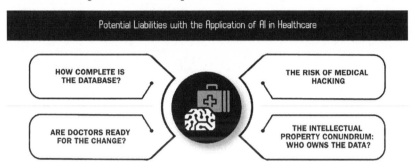

Figure 2-4. Potential liabilities with application of AI in healthcare

1. How Complete is the Database?

We must evaluate whether the raw data used to derive a conclusion is equally representative of all ethnicities and patient populations or whether it is biased toward a certain population. Precision medicine could be at risk of bias if the data did not include minority groups. In situations like this, how accurate would the analysis be if the data set provided at the source is flawed? AI may be objective, but it is not perfect. This is because of the methodology used in developing these algorithms. They not only need an abundance of information to perform analysis but also require developers to make such processes objective. Human developers are often influenced by their personal biases and may unintentionally manipulate data. This is a limitation in the development of AI in the medical world.

2. Are Doctors Ready for the Change?

The strongest resistance to the incorporation of AI into routine healthcare workflows has been from physicians who believe that the technology will eventually replace them. While the adoption of AI in healthcare is still in its nascent phase, most experts agree that its success in healthcare is due to the adjuvant efforts from healthcare professionals and that it is always the combination of technological intelligence and human intervention that brings about the best results.

Recht and colleagues[27] provide a nuanced opinion that AI may become a part of the radiology workflow by performing routine tasks like segmentation or counting, thereby enabling radiologists to perform value-added tasks like integrating clinical features with imaging reports for diagnosis while playing a critical role in integrated physician teams within healthcare systems. *Karches*[28] also maintains, "Human physician judgment will remain better suited to the practice of primary care despite anticipated advances in AI technology."

3. The Risk of Medical Hacking

Do we have the infrastructure to effectively protect and store data while maintaining patient privacy through robust encryption of medical data?

AI may be considered a double-edged sword that may be used for defense or offense, depending on the hands manning the controls. **The Future of Humanity Institute published a report on the Malicious Use of Artificial Intelligence**[29], explaining that AI-enabled tools are similar to drones that can be used to drop both medicines and bombs, leading to dynamically opposing results.

4. The Intellectual Property Conundrum: Who Owns the Data?

Healthcare is a business, and the economic gains that can be made through the correct application of AI-enabled tools in the industry could prove to be significant. It is therefore important to determine who owns this valuable data set on which AI software is applied—the data set that serves as a base for training of the algorithm, that serves to set the AI's definitions of normal so that it can then diagnose what is abnormal. Does it belong to the individual patient? To the public as a whole? To the government healthcare body that utilizes the software? Or to the private technology companies that develop the software?

Conclusion

At present, we are witnessing a meteoric rise in AI-based applications within the healthcare industry that encompasses every aspect of the patient's journey through a complex healthcare system worldwide, including consultations, symptom checking, investigations, diagnostics, and management with targeted therapeutics. The reason for the rapid adoption is the simplicity that it brings to patients, doctors, and hospital administrators. Its mimicry of human cognitive functions has enabled it to seamlessly duplicate human interventions in a field that is notorious for its intricacies and person-driven processes.

As with most novel technologies, artificial intelligence also brings its own challenges to the forefront. It raises the question of patient privacy, data security, and transparency as well as accountability if diagnosis or treatment modalities go wrong and result in poor patient outcomes. The next step in the AI journey in the healthcare industry is standardization. To ensure that technical quality and diagnostic accuracy are maintained with the applications that are actively used in patient care, a rigorous approval process is recommended. This must be delicately balanced, as too much red tape would invariably stifle the creativity with which AI designs are applied in a versatile and ever-changing field like healthcare. The US FDA has recently begun work on a new regulatory framework that aims to promote the cautious, safe, and effective development of AI-backed medical devices.[30]

There is no doubt that AI can be the defining technology of the near future. It requires clinicians with vision working alongside technical experts to set up the organizational design and the processes needed to establish an integrated and cohesive AI-enabled healthcare network. Only when the end-users work actively with the developers of the technology will AI be widely implemented to get teams out of their silos and working together.

In the words of Dr. Paul Weber[31], Associate Dean of Medical Education at Rutgers Medical School, New Jersey, USA, "We're able to train machines to exhibit human-like intelligence and apply that in a clinical setting. We haven't achieved human intelligence, but we're getting close to it."

References/Further Reading

Go to URL ⬇	Scan with a
MedMantra.com/a1	smartphone camera

CHAPTER THREE

AI-AUGMENTED HEALTHCARE – CURRENT STATE AND FUTURE APPLICATIONS

There's a new doctor in the exam room, one without a face, a name, or an identity. Artificial intelligence made a whirlwind entry into healthcare, taking many by surprise. While there is a new generation of healthcare workers who see AI as a natural progression of the rapid evolution of technology, there are industry stalwarts who believe that patient care and the human touch may be replaced by machines and robots. This mixed reception has led to the belief that it's man versus machine, prompting an in-depth look into both sides of the theory. Is AI the positive disruptor it has been proclaimed to be … or is mankind putting too much faith in a machine? Do the rewards actually outweigh the risks?

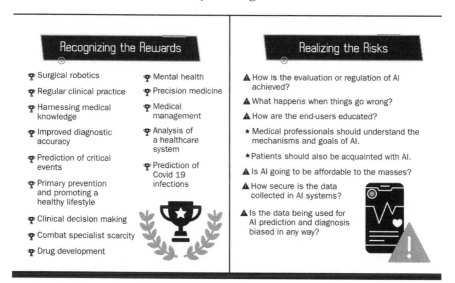

Recognizing the Rewards

- Surgical robotics
- Regular clinical practice
- Harnessing medical knowledge
- Improved diagnostic accuracy
- Prediction of critical events
- Primary prevention and promoting a healthy lifestyle
- Clinical decision making
- Combat specialist scarcity
- Drug development
- Mental health
- Precision medicine
- Medical management
- Analysis of a healthcare system
- Prediction of Covid 19 infections

Realizing the Risks

- How is the evaluation or regulation of AI achieved?
- What happens when things go wrong?
- How are the end-users educated?
- Medical professionals should understand the mechanisms and goals of AI.
- Patients should also be acquainted with AI.
- Is AI going to be affordable to the masses?
- How secure is the data collected in AI systems?
- Is the data being used for AI prediction and diagnosis biased in any way?

Figure 3-1. Recognizing the rewards and realizing the risks

Recognizing the Rewards

Deep learning, or machine learning, can significantly impact the fields where enormous data is available. The large volume of healthcare data has made the implementation of AI in this field a dream come true. The industry generates a large amount of information daily. The use of technological advancements to categorize, centralize, and stratify this data to ensure that it is both easy to access and easy to understand and interpret has been a long-standing requirement. AI can develop its own "logic" and can be used to empower healthcare personnel in an integrated medical system.

AI-enabled systems have the ability to flawlessly mimic human cognition, and the triumphs have dominated the rhetoric, both in the scientific community and the patient audience in general. AI has also helped in the integration of statistical analysis, rapid and accurate diagnosis even when applied to critical health conditions. Known as the "stethoscope of the 21st century," artificial intelligence has become the center of attraction for many specialists. In many hospitals, physicians are overburdened with a multitude of tasks, both administrative and clinical, and they find it difficult to concentrate on other procedures. That is why the technological stethoscope is making all the difference in the medical world.

Beyond administrative drudge work, the applications of AI are numerous and diverse. Nowadays, finely tuned technological robots and robust algorithms for diagnosis are making their way through the branches of medicine.

A. Surgical Robotics

In the field of surgical robotics, AI has allowed some semi-automated repetitive tasks to be undertaken by specific robots, thus increasing the efficiency of the process. An inability to exactly mimic body motion and human intelligence seems to be the drawback of robotics, which is being tackled by introducing applications like natural language processing, neural networking, speech recognition, and image recognition.

In recent times, *the Da Vinci robot* has demonstrated its success as a surgical robot, an extension of a human surgeon, who, with the aid of a console, controls the device/robot.[1,2]

Microsure is a spin-off company of the Eindhoven University of Technology and the Maastricht University Medical Center, which designed a robot to perform microsurgeries with precision.[3] The robot is controlled by a surgeon, whose hand movements are sensed and converted into tiny, accurate, and more precise movements executed by a set of "robot hands." The robotic system is augmented by AI, which is used to eliminate any tremors in the surgeon's hands, ensuring that the surgery takes place correctly.

B. Regular Clinical Practice

In regular clinical practice, basic AI systems or computer algorithms available today can be successfully employed for automating routine functions such as:

Alerts and reminders: This spans from the basic scanning of laboratory results to drug orders and the updating of the patient with scheduled reminders. Nonetheless, more advanced AI can interface with a patient monitor and detect changes in the condition of illness.[4]

Therapy pre-planning: This is specifically for conditions that require elaborate treatment plans. The patients get the advantage of receiving formulated plans that can improve their medical condition. Physicians can benefit from this as well.

Retrieval of information: Complex medical applications can be fitted with software search agents. These agents are more efficient than several web-crawling agents of the present day. To a large extent, the retrieval of information and upgrading of data is made easy.

C. Harnessing Medical Knowledge

The medical field has an ocean of knowledge that no doctor can churn up, and that, too, is growing at a more incredible pace. The doubling time of medical knowledge was fifty years in 1950, seven years in 1980, and only 3.5 years in 2010. In 2020, it was estimated to double in just seventy-three days, while training a doctor requires an arduous five-year course and a decade more for specialist training. An AI system can assist physicians by providing up-to-date medical knowledge from research journals, textbooks, and years of clinical practices across the globe to augment proper patient care. Furthermore, an AI system can extract information from an extensive patient database to make real-time reasoning for medical risk alerts and health outcome prediction.

D. Improved Diagnostic Accuracy

Diagnosis in Radiology

In the AI world, "complex" is just another word for "simple." AI has successfully eliminated issues occurring during certain angiograms and MRI scans. They can be instantaneously detected by image recognition and interpretation methods. This has attracted a significant amount of usage in many radiology clinics across the world.

Seattle-based ATL Ultrasound, Inc., made the imaging and monitoring of cardiac tissue structures simpler by developing different diagnostic ultrasound systems. The mechanism aims to eliminate irrelevant frequencies in returned signals. An adaptive intelligence algorithm is utilized to optimize many parameters when a patient is examined.[5] *Agilent Technologies in Andover, Massachusetts,* has successfully developed a smart ECG that can estimate the probability of acute cardiac ischemia (ACI).

In *John Radcliffe Hospital in Oxford*, a system was built to diagnose several heart diseases.[6] This AI diagnostic system was discovered to give about 80% accuracy compared to that of human doctors.

By using *InferVision*[7], diagnosis of illnesses and the reading of CT and X-ray scans have been made easier.

Medical Sieve is an algorithm launched by IBM to act as a cognitive assistant.[8] With its wide range of clinical know-how, it can offer analytical and reasoning solutions for the team. This technology can make sound clinical judgments in cardiology and radiology. In radiology, it can analyze images to detect problems with more efficiency and reliability.

Diagnosis in Pathology

Implementation of deep learning algorithms to whole-slide histopathology images can drastically improve diagnostic accuracy and efficiency. With AI augmentation, not only did pathologists' cancer diagnostic accuracy improve from a mere 73% to greater than 95%, but the time required to reach diagnosis decreased, too.[9] *IBM's intelligent system, Watson,* took ten minutes to interpret data of tumor cells.[10] When human doctors carried out the procedure, they spent about six days and ten hours making reasonable contributions from the genetic data. This also included the process of providing treatments and recommendations from their inferences.

A *smart microscope* developed at Harvard University[11] detects harmful infections of the blood. This AI-assisted tool was trained by treating about 25,000 slides with dye to increase the bacteria's visibility, after which about 100,000 images were pooled together. This system's total accuracy was measured at 95% − a figure surpassing that of resident doctors.

Neuromedical Systems, Inc., in New Jersey, came up with a method that is useful in screening cancer by scanning Pap smears and applying neural networks to review cells during the screening process.[12] *SkinVision* may be used for the detection of skin cancer[13] by recognizing moles and skin lesions.

E. Clinical Decision Making

Symptom checkers can track the progression or regression of chronic illnesses. Users can input their electronic health record (EHR) forms and attach additional reports such as ECGs or radiographs and get an online consultation within minutes. The benefit offered goes both ways. Physicians also get ample time to attend to more critical and emergent cases and let the app manage the rest of them.[14]

An example of such an app is Akira. In Toronto, a health tech company developed this "doctor-in-your-pocket" app to help users engage in virtual chats with their assigned healthcare providers. In this app, a patient can obtain a sick note that helps save the time required to travel to a doctor. Also, professionals can refer their patients to specialists via the app.[15]

F. Prediction of Critical Events

Using predictive analytics, artificial intelligence models can look at a patient's past medical records and find specific patterns to anticipate the patient developing a particular illness like cancer. Medical practitioners can analyze this information and get back on track, preventing their patients from developing heart attacks, diabetes, and other life-threatening ailments.

Diabetic retinopathy is the leading cause of blindness in the 21st century and can be diagnosed earlier with deep learning algorithms. Also, AI could do more with the help of the same retinal images taken for retinopathy. There are things that humans didn't quite know to look for in retinal scans, but the deep learning algorithms offered more insight into those. AI can extract information from the same eye scan, which predicts a five-year risk of having a life-threatening cardiovascular event, i.e., a heart attack or stroke.[16] This could be the basis of a newer, non-invasive way to detect cardiovascular diseases.

At the University of Nottingham, a study was published to back up this possibility.[17] A self-taught AI system was able to predict cardiovascular occurrences in some patients. Leading by a margin of accuracy of about 7.6%, the AI system had been trained on extensive data from nearly 380,000 patients. The degree of accuracy was revealed to be better than that of standard healthcare centers. The "Human Diagnosis Project" is an AI system that combines doctors' real-life experiences with machine learning.[18] Also called "Human Dx," the system's makers compile data from different healthcare centers in more than 80 countries. This covers a total of 500 institutions and 7,500 doctors. It has been said that the system will be capable of making highly accurate medical decisions and deliberations.

G. Primary Prevention and Promoting a Healthy Lifestyle

The increasing number of consumer wearables, such as the *Apple Watch* that can do quick ECG, and other medical devices combined with AI, are also being used to oversee early-stage heart diseases, enabling physicians and other caregivers to better monitor the health of patients and detect potentially life-threatening episodes at more treatable stages.[19] Another application, *Morpheo,* can be used for the detection of sleep disorders[20] by providing rich tracking data about sleep patterns.

H. Combat Specialist Scarcity

A worldwide shortage of radiologists is causing increased morbidity and mortality due to delays in diagnosis, mostly among cancer patients.[21] Researchers at the Artificial Intelligence Research Centre for Neurological Disorders, Beijing Tiantan Hospital, Beijing, developed BioMind, a Chinese AI that beat a team of top Chinese radiologists in rapidly and accurately diagnosing brain tumors.[22]

The combined skills of AI and radiologists can create a hybrid intelligence that could lead to better diagnostic accuracy and higher safety standards. AI systems could also serve as effective decision support backups, facilitating diagnoses and reducing physician burnout.

Babylon has developed an app that scans your symptoms for possible differential diagnoses, asks interactive questions to narrow down the searches, and refers you to a specialist or starts a video conference with a general practitioner right inside the app. This is literally a "Pocket Doctor" accessible to far-flung areas of the world – a step forward in bringing expert diagnosis to places where trained doctors are scarce.[14]

I. Drug Development

According to the California Biomedical Research Association, it takes an average of twelve years for a drug to reach patients who are in dire need of treatment. Only five out of 5,000 drugs that begin preclinical testing ever make it to human testing and only one of these five drugs is approved for human usage. Furthermore, it costs a company a minimum of US \$359 million for research to develop a new drug.[23]

AI frameworks are helping researchers to streamline the drug discovery and repurposing processes. AI reduces the time taken to market new drugs and significantly cuts the money invested in the development of drugs.

The creation or discovery of new drugs using AI technology requires more research and funds. If both factors were constant, AI would make a significant impact in the healthcare industry. More so, the limit of medical innovations would be infinite. Atomwise uses a database of molecular structures with supercomputers and programmed algorithms to uncover therapies. They launched a search online to virtually discover safe and existing medications that had the potential to be re-engineered for the treatment of the Ebola virus.

The company's AI technology found two drugs that were predicted to be capable of reducing the infectivity of Ebola. The best part of this is that the analysis took less than 24 hours to complete, whereas human intervention would probably take months, if not years.[24]

J. Mental Health

Cogito Corp. is a company that has improved its customer service interactions by integrating AI-powered voice recognition and analysis. *Cogito Companion*[25], the company's venture into the mental healthcare space, is an app that helps track behavioral patterns. By turning on location, the app can determine whether a patient is in their home. Communication logs make it possible to know if the patient is in touch with people. The company has said that the app does not reveal the identity of the caller. The patient's active and passive behavioral signals are monitored. If the patient has a care team, this team can monitor reports that indicate a change in the patient's overall mental health.

"Audio check-ins" are analyzed by an ML (machine learning) algorithm. Simply called voice recordings, the check-ins are akin to an audio diary. The algorithm picks up emotional cues from the audio. Characteristic voice properties that distinguish one human from another are intonation, energy, and dynamism in a conversation. Humans train this algorithm to differentiate between a "competent" and "trustworthy" sound.

They may also train the algorithm to identify a depressed patient's tone and differentiate it from that of a manic bipolar patient who is depressed. Patients can sufficiently track their moods with such real-time information, whereas healthcare practitioners can track patients' health progress. It can be seen that AI can understand human conversation facets and the mental health aspect of humans.

K. Medical Management

The first virtual nurse is known as *Molly*. A medical start-up called Sensely developed this AI nurse. With a friendly face and a pleasant voice, she monitors the health conditions and treatment of subscribers. The machine learning module offers support to patients with chronic conditions while they are getting regular treatments from doctors. *Molly* has a strong focus on chronic diseases, and it provides customized monitoring and follow-up care.[26]

Like Molly, there is *AiCure,* which monitors the frequency with which patients take their medications. Patients who find it challenging to follow medical prescriptions and advice have found the best use for this app. Endorsed by the National Institutes of Health, *AiCure* uses a webcam (on a smartphone) coupled with AI to confirm if a patient adheres to prescriptions and thereby supports patients in managing their health conditions.[27]

L. Precision Medicine

Genetics and genomics tend to be positively impacted by artificial intelligence. This is why *Deep Genomics* was created. This app finds mutations and linkages to diseases by identifying similar patterns in a database of genetic information. In due time, some systems will inform doctors about the consequences of the alteration in genetic variation – be it therapeutic or natural.

M. Analysis of a Healthcare System

In the Netherlands, over 90% of healthcare invoices are digitized. The hospital, healthcare provider, and treatment can be contained in the data. To mine this data, *Zorgprisma Publiek* Company uses IBM's Watson in the cloud to analyze invoices.[28] This company helps hospitals improve their healthcare practices. Also, patients who are unnecessarily hospitalized are well-taken care of. However, primarily, the company detects repetitive mistakes made in a clinic when treatments are administered.

N. Prediction of COVID-19 Infections

To tackle the COVID-19 global pandemic, The COVID Symptom Study, a smartphone application that was previously named the COVID Symptom Tracker, was launched in the US and the UK. Considering the large number of COVID patients who complained of loss of smell and taste, researchers wanted to use the app to determine if this symptom was specific to COVID-19. Data donated by 2,618,862 individuals were analyzed using an AI algorithm, which analyzed combinations of presenting symptoms to predict the probability of infection, which narrowed down the possibilities to 805,753. They then predicted that 140,312 out of the total participants, or 17.42% of them, were likely to be infected with COVID-19. The analysis also identified four major symptoms, which included loss of smell or taste, a cough that was dry, persistent, and severe, muscular fatigue or body pain, and loss of appetite. A total of 18,401 participants underwent a SARS-CoV-2 test, and it was revealed that 65% of those who tested positive for COVID-19 had experienced the loss of smell and taste, as opposed to only 21.7% of those who had a negative test. Considering the strong correlation between the symptoms and the disease, researchers think that this may help to provide rapid screening and diagnosis in populations who don't have access to widespread testing, although a major limiting factor is that the data is mainly self-reported and could be open to bias.[29]

Realizing the Risks

The rising global burden of disease, mismanagement of prescriptions, absence of collaborative treatment, diagnosis of rare diseases, increasing patient traffic, and growing patient data load are vital challenges in the healthcare sector. While one must acknowledge the need for faster and better healthcare resources, mankind cannot throw caution to the wind, embracing AI without being aware of possible drawbacks. AI should not be integrated haphazardly – logical reasoning is for humans, not robots.

To demonstrate the potential pitfalls in machine-based learning, its effects in systems outside healthcare can be evaluated. An "AI lawyer" was launched in September 2015 by a teenage British programmer.[30] This bot successfully helped people appeal their parking tickets. When the parking tickets are received, this bot sorts out what to do with them by asking relevant questions. Ten months after the launch, about 250,000 parking tickets had been appealed in New York and London. The success rate was penned only as 64%. In a field as sensitive as healthcare, is that success rate good enough?

Another potential area for improvement is the fact that AI researchers sometimes design the systems without keeping the end-user's comfort in mind. When evaluating the retail industry, for example, people who use eBay do not call it "AI for shopping"; it is called eBay for a reason: to appeal to the needs of the consumer so seamlessly that they don't even realize that they are using an AI-based software.

Just as every complex machine carries a description for use, the pooled information reduces the complexities of AI and the logical patterns obtained from data interpretation. Another machine cannot do this. Because AI is human-made, the operational understanding is transferred from humans to machines. This gives rise to questions that need to be asked, like:

A. How is the Evaluation or Regulation of AI Achieved?

The evaluation process is the only way the technologies' real potential can be determined for future purposes. Before an AI system is certified for diverse applications, it is subjected to a thorough analysis, one in which all processes are well documented and identified.[31]

This opens up Pandora's box of questions. How do we plan to evaluate and attach credibility to the AI software that works? Should all AI be approved? What is the vetting process? Who decides what can be used clinically? What are the benchmarking norms?

Published and released by the United States Food and Drug Administration (FDA) in January 2021, the "Artificial Intelligence/ Machine Learning (AI/ML)-Based Software as a Medical Device (SaMD) Action Plan" attempts to provide a holistic and well-rounded approach to AI-based systems by providing oversight based on lifecycle regulation. The plan aims to outline ways to support the development of "Good Machine Learning Practices" to evaluate, standardize, and improve algorithms that are based on AI. This is similar to the good practices currently existing in software engineering and quality systems. Advocating transparency to end-users fosters a patient-centered approach while boosting confidence in the idea of AI-enabled services through the advancement of real-world performance monitoring pilots.

The establishment of a total product lifecycle (TPLC) to provide oversight of AI/ML-based applications will have to be supported by the collection and monitoring of real-world data. This will allow manufacturers to figure out how their products are being used, identify the scope for improvements, and react proactively to make their products safer or more user-friendly.

This again raises a plethora of concerns for uniformity in data collection, like what type of reference data would be considered appropriate in measuring the performance of AI/ML in the field or what kind of oversight should be performed by the stakeholders. How much data is enough, and how often should the information be shared with the governing agency? What are the steps to standardize, validate and test algorithms, models, and claims by AI-supported device companies, and how should user feedback be collected and incorporated into the end design?

These standards introduced by the FDA have not been combined into a single document or provided with a robust legal framework. This gives rise to another challenge because "AI regulation" involves ethical, technical, and security-based issues, which are otherwise tackled through many different legal avenues and may differ from country to country.[32]

Validating healthcare systems that use AI is still an issue that is largely unresolved and therefore raises many questions. The goal of these regulations or standards is to ensure that the systems are safe, accurate, and precise enough for both physicians and their patients to use them with confidence.

A surprising discovery made by researchers led by the University of Cambridge revealed that out of around 300 COVID-19 machine learning AI-based models described in 2020, none have proven to be suitable for the detection or diagnosis of COVID-19 from medical imaging like chest X Rays or CT scans. This is due to flaws in methodology, biases, lack of reproducibility, and "Frankenstein datasets." These were considered to be a major weakness, considering the urgency with which COVID-19 models are needed.

"However, any machine learning algorithm is only as good as the data it's trained on," said first author Dr. Michael Roberts from Cambridge's Department of Applied Mathematics and Theoretical Physics. "Especially for a brand-new disease like COVID-19, it's vital that the training data is as diverse as possible because, as we've seen throughout this pandemic, there are many different factors that affect what the disease looks like and how it behaves."[33]

B. What Happens when Things Go Wrong?

In Montreal in 2010, a surgical operation took place by robots. The robot anesthesiologist (called McSleepy) teamed up with the surgical robot to conduct the first in-tandem performance. "The DaVinci allows us to work from a workstation operating surgical instruments with delicate movements of our fingers with a precision that cannot be provided by humans alone," said Dr. A. Aprikian, MUHC urologist in chief and Director of the MUHC Cancer Care Mission. Both doctors were widely commended for their stellar performance throughout the procedure.[34]

Five years later, a retrospective analysis of FDA data was performed by the Massachusetts Institute of Technology (MIT).[35] The objective of this research was to ascertain the safety of robotic surgery. Due to technical malfunctions, 144 patients died, while 1,391 patients sustained injuries during the study period. However, it was said that many procedures yielded results and were without problems. At the same time, complex surgical procedures such as gynecology recorded a high number of events. This incident does question the ability of surgical robots to replace human physician conducted procedures, presently.

It also highlights the missing piece of the puzzle- accountability. Who or what is responsible if things go sideways? This technology is recent, and litigation against robots hasn't been considered extensively. Thus, this is still a gray area. When a physician neglects some procedures or violates standards of care, it is regarded as medical malpractice. Theoretically, AI lacks awareness of the concept of negligence. For the robot to be held responsible for some performance standards, the existence of this standard is fundamental.

Thus, who takes the blame when the robot is unsuitable? Will the surgeon in charge of the robot be held responsible? Maybe the manufacturer of the robot? Or is it the design engineer who should be charged?

C. How are the End-users Educated?

AI will not become a reality if the fears and doubts surrounding its development are not addressed. The world needs to know the benefits and risks of this technology. Some people believe that AI can be so sophisticated that the human race will become extinct. Others fear that AI may overtake the control of our lives. Both Stephen Hawking and Elon Musk, stellar scientists, have predicted that full AI may spell doom for the human race. There must be a concerted effort to reach out and educate people about the real-life benefits of AI in healthcare in order to allay these fears.

Medical professionals should understand the mechanisms and goals of AI.

Without the support of physicians on the field, large-scale implementation of AI will be difficult in the years to come. Like with all things, the fear and apprehension of the unknown are more than likely the causes of the reluctance to embrace the benefits of AI.

An international study surveyed 1,041 radiologists and radiology residents and found that "fear of replacement and lack of adequate knowledge about the applications of AI significantly affected the perception and therefore the adoption of AI in medical professionals. 48% of radiologists and residents have an open and proactive attitude towards AI, while 38% fear replacement by AI." The authors have suggested that AI be incorporated into the training curriculum so that medical professionals are aware of it as they enter practice, and it could lead to more proactive clinical adoption.[36]

Patients should also be acquainted with AI.

Research conducted by the Harvard Business Review indicates that patients are hesitant to use health care services provided by medical artificial intelligence even when it has proven to outperform human physicians. Patients believe that their medical needs are unique and cannot possibly be addressed successfully by algorithms. Manufacturers of these AIs, such as IBM, Google, Facebook, and Baidu, should communicate effectively and transparently with the general public about AI's advancement – including the benefits and risks, to overcome the public's misgivings.[37]

D. Is AI Going to be Affordable to the Masses?

Data must be readily available for AI technologies to correctly train models, but extracting patient data from charts, reports, radiographs, and handwritten notes is cumbersome and showcases technical infrastructural deficits. The significant initial capital expenditure required to purchase the expensive clinical robotic surgical systems is a big drawback in its early adoption by the medical community. Most of the systems require the construction of new infrastructure. Also, the cost necessary to acquire the highly paid and highly skilled surgeons proficient in robotics seems to be a considerable hindrance. In order to effectively revolutionize healthcare, AI should be made available to everyone – ordinary people and not just the scientific community or those who can afford it.

E. How Secure is the Data Collected in AI Systems?

User-generated data and medical data are the bedrock of AI algorithms. However, studies have shown that the younger generation of patient populations are reluctant to share their data with large corporations.

According to the recently published FDA guidelines[32], the responsibility of data security issues while using AI algorithms would lie with the AI systems administrator (AI Officer). If these regulations are applied, it may go a long way in assuring the end-users about the security of their information, knowing that they can hold a human being accountable.

F. Is the Data Being Used for AI Prediction and Diagnosis Biased in any Way?

AI solutions have brought into the forefront a completely new criterion in the evaluation of intelligent technology: non-discrimination and equality in treatment provided. Because most medical data is recovered from electronic health records, fed and imported by human minds, it may introduce evaluation criteria that are discriminatory, even though it may be unintentional on the part of the data provider. This bias may be based on traits like ethnicity, race, or gender. The recent FDA guidelines[32] state that the data used to train the AI-based systems needs to be examined and evaluated in detail to ensure that it does not have filters that feed into this bias and adequately represent the patient population it is meant to help.

Conclusion

While it is incredibly tempting to dive headfirst into AI as a potential replacement for physicians in healthcare, as the old saying goes, we have miles to go before we sleep! AI has demonstrated its efficacy in augmenting healthcare services to a large extent; however, there are obstacles that need to be overcome, fine lines that need to be ironed out before complete implementation. Does AI actually excel on the basis of accuracy? If it were to replace doctors, what would be the unique or specific contributions it would make that could outweigh the potentially harmful effects that it could render in the medical world?

References/Further Reading

Go to URL

MedMantra.com/a2

Scan with a
smartphone
camera

CHAPTER FOUR

ARTIFICIAL INTELLIGENCE AND NEURAL NETWORKS

Thousands of real-world problems are getting solved by the new powerful artificial intelligence (AI) based techniques, which are machine learning (ML), deep learning (DL), artificial neural networks (ANNs), etc. The application of associated algorithms and AI techniques has gained remarkable popularity. The terms associated with AI may be somewhat complex and technical due to the combination of computing, electronic signal processing, mathematics, machine learning, linguistics, psychology, and most importantly, neuroscience.

In as much as this concept seems very technical, this chapter aims to break it down to such a level that rookies in the world of technology can understand it. Even non-practitioners can relate to a certain level. The main objective of this chapter is to ensure that certain complicated areas in this field of study are better understood by a good number of the masses.

Artificial Intelligence (AI) means the ability of machines to perform tasks like those performed by human intelligence. AI is a branch of computer science which deals with stimulating intelligent behavior in computers. It consists of two different types, general and narrow. General AI can perform like human intelligence and can do all tasks in all areas like a human being. Narrow AI has the ability similar to or better than human intelligence but limited to one particular area or task (like recognizing images and nothing else).

ML is a field of study that gives computers the ability to learn without being explicitly programmed (Arthur Samuel, 1959).[1] ML is a subset of AI [see Figure 4-1]. ML involves "training" a computer software algorithm (collection of commands/rules/codes) by giving it large amounts of data and then allowing it to adjust itself so that it can learn and improve its accuracy and efficiency.

ML can be divided into two main fields: Conventional (or sometimes called shallow) and deep ML. So, DL is a subset of machine learning. As of today, there is no clear definition of the term "shallow learning" in ML, as opposed to DL, which refers to automatic learning from data using artificial neural networks. Practically, DL and ANNs are interrelated, DL would not exist without ANNs, and DL and ANNs have revolutionized the field of AI. That's the reason DL and ANNs are given significant importance when it comes to the topic of AI. DL mimics the working of the human brain in processing data for a variety of use cases.

Generally, AI is referred to as the whole system which can do a specific task. ML usually works with numerical data arranged in rows and columns. DL is more flexible with data; it can work with images, text, numerical data, voice, etc.

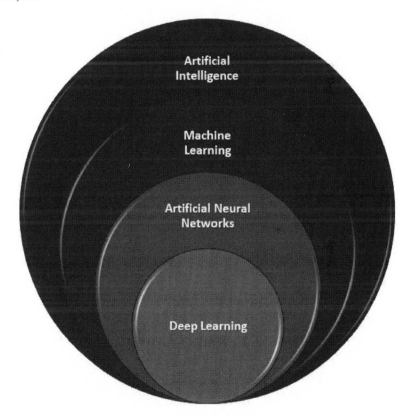

Figure 4-1. Relationship between artificial intelligence, machine learning, artificial neural networks, and deep learning

Machine Learning Algorithms

Introduction

Machine learning is based on the idea that algorithms can learn from data, identify the underlying patterns, and make decisions based on it with minimum human help. ML algorithms help recognize patterns in existing databases to predict or classify data.[2] New insights into these patterns can be made using mathematical models. It's not a new concept, but it's the one that has gained fresh momentum. With technological advancements in computational power, the rise of the internet, and smartphones, machine learning researchers got everything they dreamt of. These advancements led to the development of technologies that are applicable in almost every field.

All we need is data

The essential prerequisite for learning systems and corresponding algorithms are sufficient computing capacity and access to vast amounts of data. They are indispensable for the training of algorithms and modeling. Data can be images, words, clicks, speech, numbers, etc., whatever we can store digitally. "Big Data" has helped solve a lot of problems regarding data storage, transfer, and handling, and leveraging cloud services. We can use machine learning models on devices like smartphones, IoT (internet of things) devices with very little computational power when compared to the big servers with powerful hardware.

Despite not being recent technologies, ML and AI have significant practical importance. We use AI and ML technologies every day in our lives, knowingly or unknowingly. This applies to many areas of life and business. Internet users have benefited from this technology for long without even thinking about algorithms that work in the background. The areas of application are diverse. Consider spam detection, content personalization, document classification, sentiment analysis, customer churn forecast, email classification, upselling opportunities analysis, traffic jam prediction, genome analysis, medical diagnostics, chatbots, and much more.

The spectrum of applications spans from film and music recommendations within private environments to enhancing marketing campaigns, customer services, and logistics pathways within the business arena. A wide range of ML methods is available, including linear regression, instance-based learning, decision tree algorithms, Bayesian statistics, cluster analysis, neural networks, deep learning, and dimensionality reduction. There is a multitude of opportunities for different industries.

Making it work

For machine learning to learn from data, it must be trained by a human. This learning process begins with a prepared data set (called training data set), which is searched for patterns and correlations by a machine learning algorithm. After completing the learning process, the trained model is evaluated on unknown data. If it performs well, it is used to make predictions; otherwise, we use different parameters (settings) and algorithms to find the best results for our task.

The development of an ML model is an iterative process often run through several times until the result has reached a certain quality. There are always development loops in practice where a person must evaluate the results from the machine learning algorithm.

Machine Learning Approaches [see Figure 4-2]:

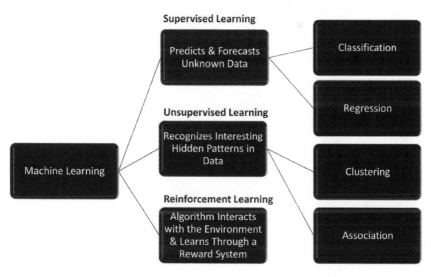

Figure 4-2. Classification of different machine learning approaches

Supervised Machine Learning

Supervised machine learning means working with labeled data. It is like telling the algorithm what pattern to look for. Like, when we watch something on YouTube, you're telling the algorithm to find similar content for you. So, it shows similar content on your home page. The model learns the mapping based on training data. In supervised learning, the relationship to a target variable is always learned, and the model tries to predict it correctly. The target variable can be a class (e.g., termination yes/no) or a numerical value (e.g., sales for the next month). The algorithm trains based on given pairs of inputs and outputs (labels). The algorithm compares the original output with the accurate output, recognizes its mistakes, and learns in this way. After that, it modifies the model accordingly. Using the model, prediction of the labels for further data that do not yet have a label can be made [see Figure 4-3].

Supervised learning is mostly used when it is possible to derive probable future events from historical data.[3] A successful learning process is used to make reliable predictions for future or unknown data. In marketing, supervised learning is often used to classify customer data. Supervised learning is very popular. Examples of supervised learning are:

- Predicting power consumption for a period of time based on past consumption

- Risk assessment in a healthcare scenario

- Prediction of failure of industrial machinery

- Forecasting customer behavior

- and many other use cases.

Unsupervised Machine Learning

The algorithm does not receive labeled data in unsupervised machine learning. It receives data from which it must independently recognize interesting and hidden groups and patterns. The fundamental difference to supervised machine learning is that unsupervised machine learning is not designed to calculate a prediction for a known target variable (e.g., classification or forecast).[4]

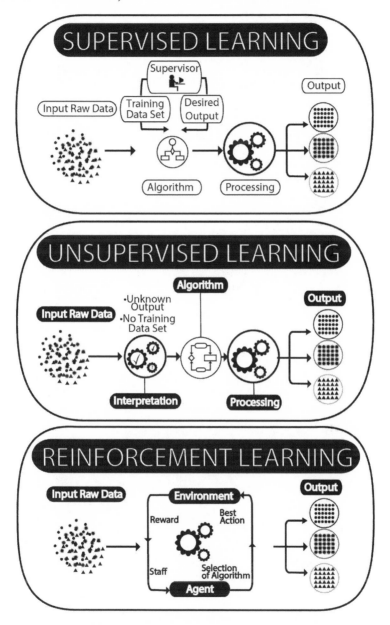

Figure 4-3. Flowcharts showing how supervised, unsupervised, and reinforcement learning works

Unsupervised ML is put into use for data without historical labels. Therefore, the system is not provided with a "correct answer." The algorithm is supposed to decode the existing data. For this purpose, the data must be examined by the algorithm for a pattern to be identified in it [see Figure 4-3 depicting unsupervised learning cycle].

Unsupervised ML can be divided into two types of problems:

Clustering: Clustering is a method of grouping objects into clusters such that objects with the most similarities remain in a group and have fewer or no similarities with objects in another group [see Figure 4-4]. Cluster analysis finds similar features amongst the data objects and groups them as per the presence or absence of these similar features.

Association: Association is a method used for finding relationships between variables in a large dataset. It determines a set of items that occurs together in the dataset. Association rule makes marketing strategy more effective. For example, people who buy X product (e.g., bread) also tend to purchase Y (butter/jam) product.

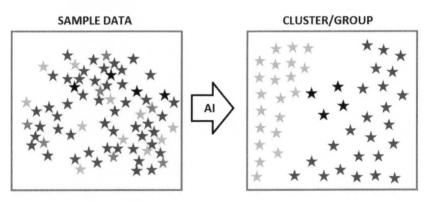

Figure 4-4. Clustering

Unsupervised learning is known to work especially well with transaction data. For example, identifying different customer groups around which to build marketing campaigns or other business strategies. Movie or YouTube video recommender systems involve grouping together users with similar viewing patterns to recommend similar content. Another real-world use case is in genetics - clustering DNA patterns to analyze evolutionary biology. Commonly used unsupervised ML algorithms include k-means clustering, k-NN (k-nearest neighbors), principle component analysis, and singular value decomposition.[5]

Partially Supervised Machine Learning

Partially supervised ML (semi-supervised ML) uses both sample data with specific target variables and unknown data and is, therefore, a mixture of supervised and unsupervised learning. The areas of application for partially supervised learning are basically the same as for supervised learning. The difference is that only a small amount of data with a known target variable is used for the learning process and a large amount where this target variable does not yet exist.[4] This has the advantage that training can be carried out with a smaller amount of labeled data. Procurement of labeled data is often extremely complex and cost-intensive. Since people often must create this data through manual processes (e.g., manual labeling of images), especially in the image or object recognition. Here a small data set of known (labeled) images is created. This is usually done by people. Then rest of the data is labeled using this model. Subsequently, for example, an artificial neural network is trained for classification and then applied to the rest of the data. This way, the sample data for the unknown data can be created correctly and quickly.

Reinforcement Learning

Reinforcement learning (RL) algorithms learn using trial and error to achieve an objective. RL consists of three parts, the agent (learner), the environment (everything the agent interacts with), and actions (what the agent does). Agent receives a reward or a penalty for its action based on the objective or the policy. The goal is to maximize rewards. The algorithm is not shown which action is the right one in which situation but instead receives positive or negative feedback from the cost function (a mechanism that returns the error between predicted outcomes and the actual outcomes). The cost function is then used to estimate which action is the right one at which point in time. Thus, the system learns "to reinforce" through praise or punishment to maximize the reward function.

The main difference from unsupervised and supervised learning is that reinforcement learning does not require sample data in advance. The algorithm can develop its own strategy in many iterative steps in a simulation environment [see Figure 4-4].

Reinforcement learning is used in robotics, computer games, and navigation. Through trial and error, the algorithm recognizes the actions that bring the greatest reward in reinforcement learning. The target of the agent is to select actions that maximize the expected reward within a specific time. The target can be achieved relatively rapidly if an appropriate strategy is employed. Learning the best strategy is the aim of reinforcement learning. Reinforcement learning is the great hope of many AI researchers for solving complex problems, such as autonomous driving, autonomous robotics, and the development of general artificial intelligence.

Autonomous vehicles use reinforcement learning to learn to drive, keeping safety first, and obeying traffic rules. The reinforcement learning agent (algorithm) learns from the system of rewards and penalties to achieve specific goals like keeping the vehicle in lane, avoiding collision, overtaking correctly, and more. The agent interacts with (but cannot change) the environment (roads, traffic, etc.) around it.

Commonly Used Machine Learning Algorithms:

ML algorithms can be broadly classified into conventional and deep ML algorithms. All ML algorithms that are not deep are called conventional (or occasionally shallow). Examples of conventional ML algorithms include linear regression, decision tree, K-nearest neighbor, Naïve-Bayes, support vector machines, etc.

Regression

Regression is a statistical method that helps us understand the relationship between two or more variables. It helps to understand which factors are important and should be considered and which can be ignored.

Regression finds the relationship between the dependent and independent variables. The dependent variable is the factor/value which we are trying to calculate; as it depends on other factors, it is named so. Independent variables are the values/factors which influence the prediction values. Regression is of two types, linear and polynomial regression.

1. *Linear Regression*

It is one of the most versatile statistical methods. Simple linear regression is a linear regression analysis that allows for only one predictor to be considered. Here we use only one variable to predict the output. In linear regression, the regression model predicts the values for the dependent variable based on the independent variables. For example, increasing sales are observed with increasing purchasing power of the customers. Usually, increasing the dosage of an antihypertensive drug leads to decreasing blood pressure in patients, which is a linear correlation.

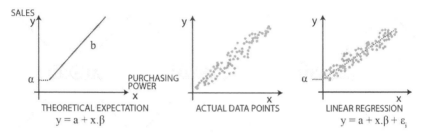

Figure 4-5. Straight-line through the data points showinglinear regression

Linear regression is represented as a straight line that, at its best, determines the relationship between the input variable 'x' and the output variable 'y'.[6] This is done by determining certain weights for the input variables that are also referred to as coefficients β, and the 'y' is predicted based on the input 'x.' The linear regression learning algorithm is aimed at the determination of the value for the coefficients. Our goal is to best fit a line that can describe the properties of data [see Figure 4-5]. We are therefore looking for a function in regression that describes our point cloud - with which we are confident that we can make predictions about the dependent variable. Here, the target value (dependent variable) is 'y, and the input value is 'x.' So, we work in a two-dimensional world. It should also be noted that a point cloud can never be perfectly described by a straight line. In a two-dimensional system (one input and one output), we speak of simple regression.

Variables that mathematically define the function are often represented as Greek letters (β, α, ε, etc.). The model describes how a series of input values (n = number of x-dimensions) and a series of weights (n + 1) results in a function that calculates a y-value. Here we use n + 1 weights as n + 1th weight is the intercept of the line. This calculation is also known as forward propagation. How do we make the forward propagation spit out the correct values? We employ backpropagation.

Backpropagation is an optimization method that uses the gradient method to calculate the error of forward propagation and adapt the weights in the opposite direction of the error. It is optimized in such a way that the error is minimized. It is an iterative process in which a forward propagation is carried out repeatedly based on training data, and with each iteration step, the prediction results are compared with the specified results (the marked training data), and the errors are thus calculated. The resulting error function is convex (U-shaped), derivable, and has a central global minimum. We find this minimum through this iterative approach. For more than 200 years, science has known linear regression, and it has been thoroughly researched. A few good rules of thumb during the usage of these methods include the removal of very similar variables (correlated) and the removal of noise from the data, if feasible. Therefore, linear regression is both a quick and easy method and an excellent first algorithm to try out.

2. *Polynomial Regression*

Polynomial regression (PR) is used to fit nonlinear relationships in data. In many cases, the relationship between the dependent and independent variables cannot be expressed appropriately through a straight line. In such cases, we use different curves to fit our data and predict better results [see Figure 4-6]. PR helps us develop flexible ML models that calculate the potential death rate by analyzing many dependent factors or variables. In COVID-19 pandemic, these variables can be pre-existing chronic diseases, living or working in crowded places, access to face masks, etc. PR is often used to monitor the spread of tumors in cancer patients, as the tumor spread often has a non-linear character. We need to use this algorithm carefully, as a wrong approach could lead to overfitting (the algorithm performs well on the given data, but in practical application, it struggles to provide proper predictions).

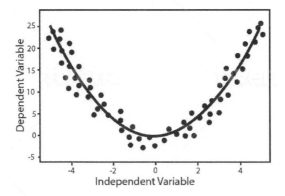

Figure 4-6. Graph of polynomial regression - a curve representing data properties

Logistic Regression

Logistic regression works where the dependent variable is categorical, i.e., data containing the only integral value to represent its class. It is used to predict whether an event or person passes or fails, wins or loses, healthy or sick, etc. It can also be extended to multi-class classification or multinomial logistic regression, where instead of two categories, dependent variables can be classified into more than two categories. It mostly deals with problems related to binary classifications (i.e., problems with two class values).

This is an alternative method that has been adopted from the field of statistics by machine learning. As with linear regression, the goal of logistic regression is the determination of the values for the coefficients that weight each of the output variables. A nonlinear function called the logistic function is used to convert the prediction for the output.[7] The logistic function resembles 'S' [see Figure 4-7]. Its task is to convert the given value into a range that is from 0 to 1. This is essential because the rule may be applied to the logistic function's output to bind the values to 0 and 1 (e.g., if the output is less than 0.5, the output is 0) and for the prediction of a class value.[4]

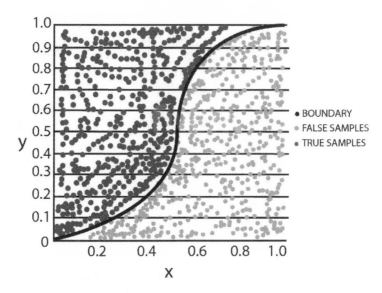

Figure 4-7. Logistic regression - 'S' shaped logistic function acting as a boundary between two classes

As the model learns, there is an option to use the logistic regression predictions as a probability for the instance of the given data assigned to either class 0 or class 1. This is particularly helpful in solving the problems where a prediction needs to be better justified. As with linear regression, logistic regression works better if both the attributes that are not related to the output variable and the attributes that are relatively very similar are eliminated. Logistic regression is, therefore, a quick model to learn. It can also solve the problems of binary classification very effectively.

When formulating the regression model, it must be decided which variables are included in the model as dependent and as independent variables. Theoretical considerations play a central role in this. The model should be kept as simple as possible. It is therefore advisable not to include too many independent variables. The ordering of independent variables also plays a significant role in logistic regression. If all independent variables are completely unrelated, then the order in which they are introduced into the model is irrelevant. However, the variables are rarely completely unrelated. The method of variable inclusion is, therefore, relevant.

With the help of logistic regression, we can make statements about the probability with which a certain form of an independent variable will be found in a condition of the dependent variable. Imagine the example of caffeine consumption and the ability to concentrate. Instead of measuring the concentration on a continuous scale from 1 to 100, you could simply ask the test subjects whether they are feeling focused or not.

Discriminant Analysis

Discriminant analysis (DA) is used to analyze problems to differentiate or discriminate data into discrete/distinct classes. For example, a physician could perform a discriminant analysis to identify patients at high or low risk for heart attack. DA can also be used in real life to differentiate between the price sensitive and non price sensitive buyers of groceries in terms of their psychological attributes or characteristics. DA contains the statistical properties of the data that are calculated for each class. It includes the following for a single variable input:

- the mean for each class

- the variance calculated for all the classes.

The predictions are made via the calculation of a discriminant value for each of the classes and making a prediction for the class that has the highest value. This method assumes that the data has a Gaussian distribution or normal distribution (bell curve) and different classes have class-specific means and equal variance/covariance. If these assumptions are violated, logistic regression will outperform Linear Discriminant Analysis (LDA). Therefore, it is recommended to eliminate the outliers from the data in advance. Discriminant analysis is best suited for tackling predictive modeling problems.

Decision Trees

A decision tree is drawn upside down with its root at the top and leaf nodes at the bottom. The tree is split into branches and edges. Trees cover both classification as well as regression-related problems. It is a flowchart-like structure, and its internal nodes denote different test conditions, the branch denotes the outcome of the test, and the last nodes (leaf nodes) hold class labels or output [see Figure 4-8].

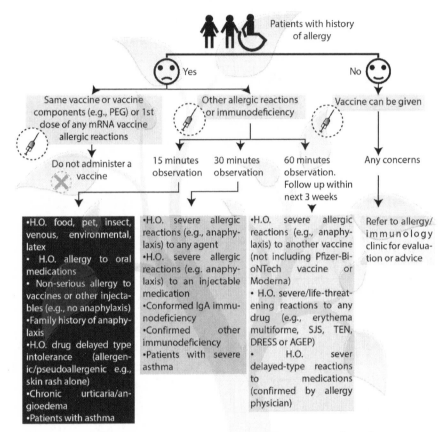

Algorithm for COVID-19 vaccination and physician response for patients with suspected allergy

Abbreviations: Erythema multiforme (EM), Stevens-Johnson syndrome (SJS), toxic epidermal necrolysis (TEN), Drug reaction with -eosinophilia and systemic symptoms (DRESS), Acute generalized - exanthematous pustulosis (AGEP). polyethylene glycol (PEG)

Figure 4-8. A decision tree contains root at the top and leaves at the bottom

A decision tree is a robust algorithm used for the predictive modeling of ML. The model of a decision tree is represented as a binary tree. A binary tree has a straightforward structure because it consists of algorithms and data structures. Each node is used to represent an individual input ('x') and a division point of this variable (provided that the variable is a numeric one). The end nodes of the tree consist of an output variable ('y') that is used in making a prediction: the tree divisions run through to the end node, and the class value is the output at the same end node. Trees are quick to learn and very quick in determining predictions. Additionally, they are often precise in solving diverse problems and do not need special preparation of the data.

One must descend along the tree from the root node to the leaf node to get a classification or output. A tree essentially contains the rules for answering only one question. In a problem with low complexity, a binary decision tree is used for prediction. Decision trees are less appropriate for predicting continuous values and are prone to errors due to the relatively small dataset.

Decision trees may either be manually written by experts or automatically deduced from gathered experience using ML techniques. There are many competing algorithms available for this. According to the top-down principle, the decision trees are mostly inferred recursively (from root to leaf nodes). For this purpose, the dataset needs to contain values using which decisions can be made. A split on the data is performed at each node based on one of the input features, generating two or more branches as output. More and more splits are done in the upcoming nodes, and increasing numbers of branches are generated to partition the original data. This continues until a node is generated where all or almost all of the data belong to the same class, and further splits or branches are no longer possible.

Ultimately, a decision tree describing the experience of the training data in formal rules is created. Now, the trees may be used for the automatic classification of other data records or for the interpretation and evaluation of the resulting set of rules.

All algorithms for the automatic induction of decision trees are based on the same recursive top-down principle. The only difference is in their criteria for the selection of the values and attributes of the rules at the nodes of the tree, in their criteria for the cancellation of the induction process, and in the likely post-processing steps that subsequently optimize a branch of a tree that has already been calculated (or entire trees) using various criteria.

A considerable benefit of the decision trees is that they are relatively easy to both understand and explain. This is especially useful when the basic properties of the data cannot be determined from the outset.

An often-mentioned drawback of the decision trees is the relatively low quality of classification when the trees are made use of for automatic classification. Because of their discrete set of rules, the trees perform somewhat worse for most real-world classification problems as compared to the other classification techniques like artificial neural networks or support vector machines. This implies that even though the trees can create easily understandable rules for people, these understandable rules often do not have the best possible quality for problem-solving in the real world. Another drawback is the possible sizes of the decision trees if no simple rule can be induced from the training data.

This can have several negative effects: on the one hand, a human viewer quickly loses the overall view of the connection between the many rules, and on the other hand, such large trees tend to lead towards over-adaptation to the training data record so that the new data records are automatically incorrectly classified. Methods were therefore developed to shorten the decision trees to a reasonable size. For instance, one may either limit the maximum depth of the trees or set in place a minimum number of objects per node.

The error rate of a decision tree is equal to the number or amount of the wrongly classified data objects relative to all the data objects in a data record. This number is determined regularly on either the training data used or, even better, on a set of data objects that are categorized as accurately as possible, disjointed from the training data, also called test data.

Depending on the area of application, it can be particularly important to keep either the false positive objects (incorrect classification of disease when no disease is present in the test subject) or the false negative objects (fails to indicate the presence of a condition when it is present) especially low. For example, in emergency medicine, it is far less harmful to treat a healthy patient than not to treat a sick patient. The effectiveness of decision trees is, therefore, always context-dependent.

Decision trees can be combined with neural networks. In this way, it is possible to replace inefficient branches of a tree with neural networks to achieve a higher classification quality that cannot be achieved with the trees alone. The advantages of both classification methods can also be used by mapping partial structures into the other methodology: The trees do not need as much training data for induction as the neural networks, and due to this, they can be quite inaccurate, especially when they're small. The neural networks, on the other hand, classify more precisely but require more training data. Therefore, one can try to use the properties of the decision trees for the generation of parts of neural networks by the so-called TBNNs (Tree-Based Neural Networks) that translate the rules of the decision trees into the neural networks.[8]

Naïve-Bayes

This is a relatively basic but astonishingly strong predictive modeling algorithm. It assumes that the presence of a particular feature in a class is unrelated to the presence of any other feature. For example, a fruit may be considered to be an apple if it is red, round, and about 3 inches in diameter. All the properties of a class contribute independently to calculating probability, and that's why it is known as 'naïve.' In other words, it means each input variable is independent. It is based on the Bayes theorem.

It calculates two kinds of probabilities:

i.   the probability of each class,

ii. the conditional probability for each class for each specified value.

These probabilities are calculated directly from the training data. After the calculation is done, the probability model is employed for the determination of the predictions for the new data utilizing the Bayes theorem. For the data that has real value, a Gaussian distribution or normal distribution (bell-shaped) is usually assumed to make the estimation of these probabilities easier.

K-Nearest Neighbors (k-NN)

This algorithm assumes that similar things exist near or in close proximity to each other. The k-NN algorithm is another basic but effective ML algorithm. It uses the entire dataset at once to calculate similar clusters of data points. To make a prediction, it tries to fit each data point into each of the clusters and finally classifies it to the best-suited one. Generally, it uses Euclidean distance to calculate the similarity between data points, but we can use several other techniques that best suit our problem. We need to tell the algorithm how many data points need to be in a cluster. This led to its naming as k-Nearest Neighbors. It puts the 'k' number of nearest points in the same cluster. It votes for the most frequent label (in classification, i.e., integers) or averages the labels (in regression, i.e., a number with decimals) as output [see Figure 4-9].

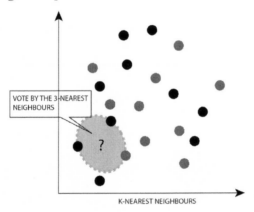

Figure 4-9. Graphical representation of k-NN showing a cluster of three nearest data points

It should also be pointed out that k-NN may require a large amount of storage space or a lot of memory to store all the data. However, this algorithm will only perform a calculation (or training) whenever there is a requirement for a prediction. If the training instances are updated and monitored over time, the predictions are kept accurate. Generally, we use the most relevant features or variables to predict the output.

For a small application, the risk is particularly great if the training data are not equally distributed or if there are only a few examples. If the training data is not evenly distributed, a weighted distance function can be used that assigns greater weight to closer points than more distant ones. A practical problem is the large storage and computing effort requirement of the algorithm with high dimensions and a lot of training data.

Genetic Algorithms (GAs)

GAs are search-based optimization techniques based on genetics and the principle of natural selection. Optimization means finding input values such that we get the best output. Generally, it refers to maximizing or minimizing a function. Genetic algorithms mimic the principle of biological evolution. To find an approximate answer to a problem of optimization, evolutionary principles such as mutation or selection are applied to the populations of solution candidates.

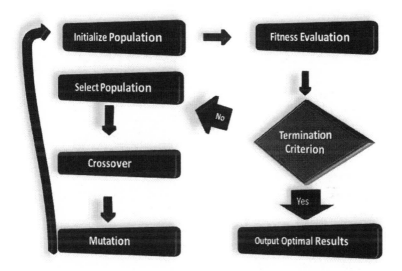

Figure 4-10. Flowchart showing a genetic algorithm

We have a pool or a population of possible solutions to the given problem. These solutions then undergo recombination and mutation (changes like in natural genetics), producing new children, and the process is repeated over various generations. Each individual (or candidate solution) is assigned a fitness value (based on its objective function value), and the fitter individuals are given a higher chance to mate and yield more "fitter" individuals. This is similar to

"Survival of the Fittest." In this way, we keep "evolving" better individuals or solutions over generations till we reach a stopping criterion. The algorithm terminates when either a maximum number of generations has been produced or a satisfactory fitness level has been reached for the population [see Figure 4-10].

Let us imagine a box with auto parts. If the box is shaken long enough, there is a chance (however small) that after a while, a roadworthy car will be assembled within the box. This random generation model makes it extremely unlikely that anything nearly complex, let alone a living organism, could arise. As we would like to further develop the population of the solution candidates, there is a requirement for a suitable representation.

The fitness function mimics the environment of biological evolution. This is often identical to the function to be optimized. A method for selecting the solution candidates according to their fitness is used for the simulation of the selection of biological evolution. A simple method is to convert fitness into a probability of selection, which is then used to decide which individuals will be transferred to the next generation without change.[9] This is repeated until we get desired results.

GAs generally perform better for real-world problems than other optimization processes like Gradient-based methods. GAs also deliver fast results that suit real-world applications.

Learning Vector Quantization (LVQ)

LVQ is a prototype-based supervised classification algorithm. It applies a winner-take-all Hebbian learning-based approach. It is a precursor to self-organizing maps (SOM) and related to the k-nearest neighbor algorithm (k-NN). It compresses data by assigning reference vectors to data points and sending only the optimum reference vectors instead of the entire data. The LVQ model is based on the similarity (or dissimilarity/distance) measure between the test object and the reference vectors, called codebook vectors or prototypes.[10] For each data point, the LVQ model, determines the prototype closest to the input. This winner prototype is then moved closer if it correctly classifies the data point or moved away if it classifies the data point incorrectly. LVQ models can be applied to multi-class classification problems, especially in classifying text documents.

Support Vector Machines (SVMs)

The function of SVMs is to find a hyperplane in N-dimensional space (N = number of features) that distinctly classifies data. A hyperplane refers to a straight line/plane that divides the input variable space. It can also be referred to as a decision boundary [see Figure 4-11]. There may exist many such hyperplanes, but our objective is to find the one with maximum margin. This may be represented in two dimensions as a straight line or as a plane in three dimensions.[11]

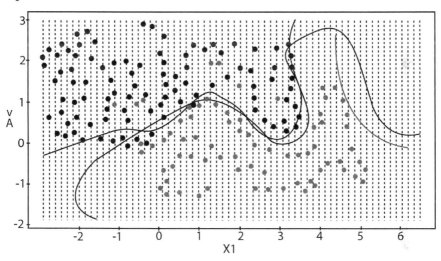

Figure 4-11. Graphical representation of a support vector machine

A vector in a vector space symbolizes each object. Support vectors are the data points that are closer to the separating hyperplane. The position of these support vectors influences the orientation of the hyperplane. We try to find the maximum separation between these support vectors and the hyperplane. The optimal or best hyperplane that can divide the two classes is a straight line that has the largest margin.

During the insertion of the hyperplane, it is not required to consider all the training vectors. The vectors that are at a greater distance from the hyperplane are 'hidden' to an extent behind the other vectors and do not affect the separation plane's position. The hyperplane is only dependent on the closest vectors, and only they are required to describe the layer precisely in a mathematical manner.

It is impossible to 'bend' a hyperplane, and so a clean separation with a hyperplane is feasible only if the objects are linearly separable. This condition is not commonly met for real sets of training objects. In most real-life datasets, data cannot be separated using a straight line. Support vector machines make use of the kernel trick to draw a nonlinear class boundary.

For such data, we apply some mathematical transformations to add more dimensions. SVMs convert non-separable problems into separable problems and are most useful in nonlinear separation problems. Now, this data can be separated using a straight line. Most of the algorithms have inbuilt features to calculate best-suited transformations, so it's not done manually. When transforming again into the lower-dimensional space, the linear hyperplane becomes a nonlinear hyperplane, possibly even a non-contiguous hyperplane that divides the training vectors cleanly into two classes—using which predictions can be made for new data points.

Bagging and Random Forest

One of the most well-known and powerful algorithms in ML is random forest. It is a type of ML ensemble algorithm that is also known as either bootstrap aggregation or bagging. An ensemble method is a technique that combines the predictions from multiple machine learning algorithms together to make more accurate predictions than any individual model.

In bootstrap, we make small groups of our original data, and then we calculate the mean of each small group and average it out. We use this average as the mean of the original data instead of calculating the mean of it directly. It can be applied to find other quantities.

Numerous samples of the training data are obtained, and models are created for each data sample. When the making of a prediction is required for new data, each of the models makes a prediction, after which each prediction is averaged to obtain a better estimate of the actual output.

A random forest is a classification procedure in which the decision trees are created in such a way that suboptimal divisions are carried out by introducing randomness instead of selecting optimal division points. The models created for each data sample, therefore, differ more than they would otherwise but are correct in their exclusive and distinctive way. Through the combination of their predictions, the true base output value is better estimated. In simple words, a large number of individual decision trees are made, and the most common answer among their predictions is selected.

Boosting

Boosting is an ensemble method for the creation of a sole good classifier from several relatively weak classifiers. For this purpose, a model is created from the training data and a second model for the improvement of the errors of the first model.[12] The peculiarity of Boosting is that the models are continually added until the ideal prediction of the training set or the addition of a maximum number of models.

It learns from the mistakes of the previous model and tries to correct them in the next model till we get good results.

Boosting is of three types:

AdaBoost (Adaptive Boosting)

It is the first successful boosting algorithm. AdaBoost uses decision trees with a single split, and these decision trees are called decision stumps. In the first decision stump, all observations are equally weighted. Incorrectly labeled decisions are weighted more than the correctly classified observations to correct errors of the previous model. It can be used for both classification and regression (predicting continuous numerical value) tasks.

The models are built one at a time and perform the task of updating the weights of the training instances, which affect the performance of the next tree in the sequence. After the creation of all the trees, the predictions for new data can be made [see Figure 4-12]. Since a lot of attention is paid to correcting errors using this algorithm, we get clean data.

Algorithm Adaboost - Example

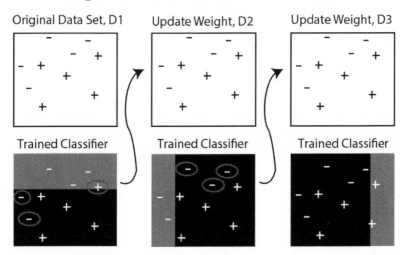

Figure 4-12: AdaBoost – the final model can classify data points more accurately

Gradient Boosting

It employs gradient descent to find the shortcomings of the previous model. Instead of changing weights for predictions, it tries to predict new values in place of erroneous values. The final model can correct a lot of errors from previous models. This leads to better results over time.

XGBoost

It stands for extreme gradient boosting. It is a library that is focused on computational speed and model performance. It supports multiple interfaces like:

- Command-line interface (CLI)

- C++

- Python

- R

- Julia

- Java and Java Virtual Machine (JVM) like Scala and Hadoop

Gradient boosting is slow due to higher computational cost. It provides Parallelization, Distributed Computing, Out-of-Core Computing, and Cache Optimization features. It is an open-source software that is available for use under the Apache-2 license.

Differences between bagging and boosting

Bagging employs parallel models, and their output is averaged according to problem type (classification or regression). Whereas in boosting, a single learner is improved over time using different approaches [see Figure 4-13].

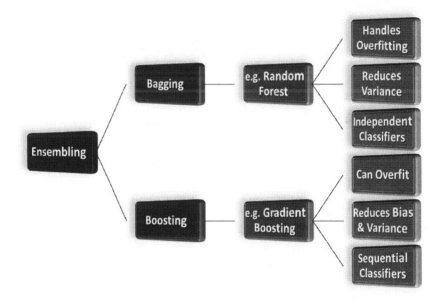

Figure 4-13. Differences between bagging and boosting

Neural Networks (NN)

Artificial neural networks are the basis of deep learning. They are inspired by the working of neurons in the human brain.

An overview of biological neural networks

To date, the most powerful computing machine ever known is the human brain. No other machine has been able to supersede its complexities. A neuron consists of a cell body from which multiple dendrites come out, along with a long tube-like axon having multiple axon terminals at its other end [see Figure

4-14]. Axon terminals are interfaces where the neurons communicate with one another, and a synapse (a gap) connects the terminals to dendrites.

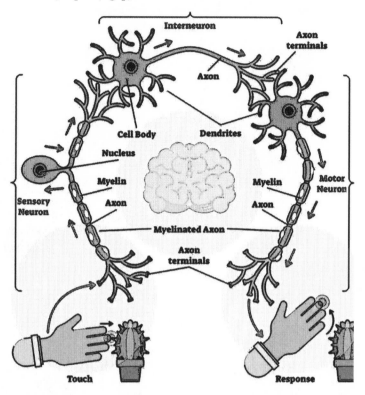

Figure 4-14. Three types of neurons, sensory neuron, interneuron, and motor neuron

A neuron, also known as a nerve cell, is an electrically excitable cell that receives, processes, and transmits information through electrical and chemical signals

© **Can Stock Photo / normaals**

A neuron in the brain can be considered to be equivalent to a tiny transistor in a computer, also called a node in the artificial neural network. The concept of neurons (brain cells) and network of neurons are the models upon which the inner workings of the human brain depend on. In fact, an estimated number of 100×10^9 neurons are contained in the human brain, with each connected through their pathways to the rest of the brain [see Figures 4-15 and 4-16].

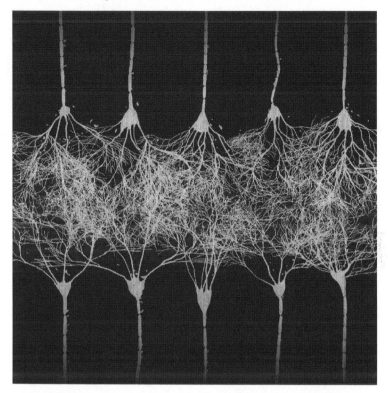

Figure 4-15. Neurons or nerve cells form a massive network

© Can Stock Photo / whitehoune

In the biological neural network, the transmission of input signals (sensory data) occurs from one layer of neurons to another through their numerous interconnections. Usually, a single neuron in the deeper layers can receive thousands of input connections, and each neuronal layer may contain a few dozen to millions of neurons.

In generating input signals, all five senses are of utmost importance. Other processes that may apply include ingestion – breathing, eating, and drinking. Before the output is delivered, multiple biochemical-physiological processes occur in the deeper neuronal layers. Then, the brain acts by instructing to act (motor signals), recollecting memory, and so on.

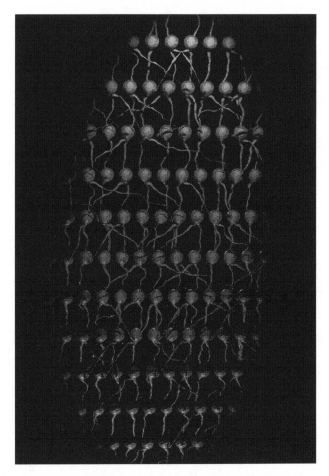

Figure 4-16. Neurons or nerve cells form a network

© Can Stock Photo / tdhster

The neural networks are the reason our brain carries out the functions of 'thinking' or 'processing' every action. As soon as our body – muscles and organs inclusive – receive the subsequent instructions from the brain, the action takes place. Nevertheless, the neural networks of the brain are capable of changing and updating by modifying their processes as a response to new learning and more experience.

If a computing machine wants to perform human-like activities, then it should replicate the functionalities and capability of the human brain. This includes intelligence. Thus, an artificial version of a network of neurons must be successfully implemented by the machine.

An overview of artificial neural networks (ANNs)

Artificial neural networks (ANNs) are algorithms that are modeled to a certain extent on the human brain. Neural networks are a very active research area and are considered the basis for artificial intelligence. They work on various data sources such as images, sound, text, tables, or time series in order to extract information and recognize patterns.

Multiple neurons in various layers of the human brain are interconnected to form massive biological neural networks. The ANNs are designed to mimic biological neural networks. The neuron or nerve cell equivalent in the ANN is called a "node." The ANNs are actually virtual or simulated networks created inside the computer software. The ANNs need not be programmed to do a particular task; they can rather be trained or learn on their own, similar to a human brain!

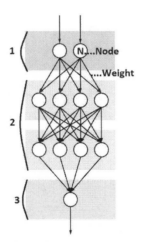

Figure 4-17: Artificial Neural Network (ANN) - an artificial network of interconnected nodes (N). Layer 1 represents the input layer, layer 2 represents the hidden layer, and layer 3 represents the output layer. Each connection between two nodes is represented by a variable number called a weight (W)

© Can Stock Photo / korolev

One or more nodes are arranged in multiple layers in a typical artificial neural network. A typical ANN has three distinct layers. These are an input layer, the hidden layers, and the output layer [see Figure 4-17]. The input layer lies at the top of the network. The hidden layers lie below the input layer, and the output layer lies at the bottom of the network. In a typical ANN, each node in the hidden and output layers is connected with each and every node in the layer above. Each connection represents a variable number called a "weight." Input layer nodes receive the data to be processed. Output layer nodes output the result(s) obtained after processing the data in the hidden layers.

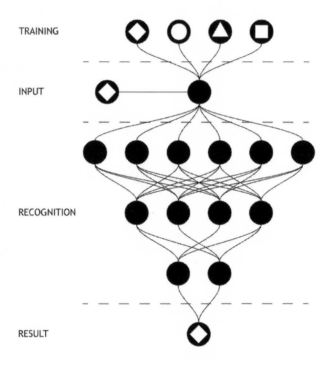

Figure 4-18. Artificial Neural Network (ANN)

© Can Stock Photo / korolev

When the ANN is being trained, the input layer nodes receive the data and pass it on to the nodes in the next hidden layer. The same thing happens when a trained ANN is performing a task it is trained to do. The input data is passed on from the input layer node(s), through the hidden layer nodes, and finally to the output layer node(s). The output layer node(s) give out the output data or the result [see Figure 4-18]. Since the data flows forward from the input to the output layer, this type of network is called a "feed-forward network." Data, in this case, is in the binary form - a matrix of numbers 0 and 1 in varying combinations. Any type of input data like an image, text, or audio is represented in the ANN in a binary form.

When the input layer has more than one node, each node receives the same input data. The number of output layer neurons is determined by the number of classes in the data. When the data passes through a connection between any two nodes, a mathematical function applies a weight (a small variable number that can either be positive or negative) to the data and modifies it. In simple terms, the mathematical function multiplies the input data value with the variable number of the connection weight and passes on the product to the node below it. Each node has a threshold value. The node adds all input data values, and if this summation value exceeds the threshold, then the node is activated and passes on the modified data to all the connected nodes in the next layer – a process called excitation.

Different connections may have different weights. During the training of an ANN, these weights need to be adjusted so that a correct result is obtained from the output layer. It has been proven that, given enough time to try to find the optimum weights for different connections, any artificial neural network can output the correct result! Various optimization techniques are used to expedite this process of finding optimum weights for various connections in an ANN, like gradient descent and stochastic gradient descent, to name a few. In fact, the current rapid and significant increase in the processing power of the graphics processing units (GPUs) has enabled us to reduce this optimization time from years/months to a few days/hours. This is one of the most important reasons why the ANNs have become practical and economical today.

While training an ANN for a given input data, our aim is to match the output data with the expected answer, as, answer to the input data (question) is already known. Without any training, the ANN may not give a correct answer. The difference in the actual output and the expected output (correct answer) is gradually reduced during training by changing the connection weights. This process of changing the connection weights is done in a reverse direction (bottom-up), starting from the output layer and gradually (layer by layer) moving up towards the input layer. This is the reason the process is called backpropagation. It is usually shortened to backprop.

During training, a sufficient number of pre-evaluated input data samples are used. Training is complete when the actual output exactly matches the expected output for all of the sample data. The connection weights present at this time remain fixed when the trained ANN is used in the future until it receives further training. This can be explained by a simple real-world example. Imagine as if we need to train an ANN to correctly recognize two distinct forms of oral medication - a capsule and a round flat tablet. In an ANN with one input node and one output node, we can assume that a capsule is represented by a 1 and the tablet by a 0 (binary digit). When training this ANN, our aim should always be to obtain an output of 1 when the input node sees a capsule and an output of 0 when the input node sees a tablet. When we start training the ANN to recognize a capsule, we feed the ANN with different images of capsules and use the above-described backpropagation method to gradually change the weights of different connections till we always obtain an output of 1. A similar process is repeated when training the ANN to recognize a tablet until we always obtain an output of 0. The fully trained ANN can then correctly recognize any type of capsule or tablet not seen by it before. The more and varied samples an ANN is trained with, the more accurate it becomes.

Shallow ANNs have very few hidden layers, while deep ANNs have a high number of hidden layers. Deeper ANNs are designed to carry out complex data recognition tasks, like identifying images and finding patterns in a large text database. In a deeper ANN, the superficial hidden layers learn to recognize simpler features and the deeper layers learn to recognize more complex features. The deeper the hidden layer, the more complex the feature it can recognize. For example, in a deep ANN trained to recognize human faces, the superficial hidden layers recognize simpler features like edges and overall shape of the face, and the deeper hidden layers recognize complex features like the size and shape of the nose, the color of the iris and the size and shape of the eyebrows, etc.

A complex ANN model [see Figure 4-19] with more efficient problem-solving ability and increased abstraction can be created by:

- Increasing the frequency of hidden layers

- Increasing the number of paths between neurons

- Increasing the number of neurons in a given layer

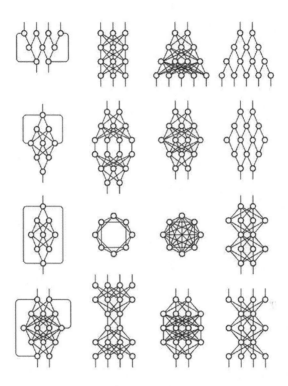

Figure 4-19. Different types of Artificial Neural Networks (ANNs)

© Can Stock Photo / korolev

However, increased model complexity is often associated with an increased chance of overfitting. Overfitting means the failure of an ANN algorithm such that it gives suboptimal results when fed unknown data but gives optimum results when fed training (previously known) data. Increased time requirements and computational resources can be consequences of complexities in model and algorithm as well.

Parallelism is the 'term' employed in modeling and processing nonlinear relationships between the input and output nodes. ANNs can be used in a lot of applications and are the important components of a broad field of machine learning.[13]

The complexity of ANNs is difficult to analyze because they are very powerful – the reason they have been termed as 'black box algorithms.' The inner workings of these algorithms have complexities that cannot be explained; finding solutions to problems by using ANN should be done, bearing this in mind.

Deep Learning (DL)

Deep learning is a subset of machine learning. It uses ANNs to learn from data. Recall that artificial neurons or processing nodes are used to transform input data throughout the different layers of an ANN. Deep learning neural networks have a greater number of hidden layers of artificial neurons and a complex architecture. The chain of transformations that occur from input to output layers is called the credit assignment path (CAP). In a deep learning model, the concept of depth is measured using the CAP value. While some scientists consider deep learning to be really deep when CAP > 10, others consider CAP > 2 as deep.[13] Shallow learning algorithms have a lesser number of hidden layers of neurons (usually a single) and are less complex as compared to deep learning algorithms.

Deep learning excels in the area of unsupervised feature extraction. Further learning, understanding, and generalization are made by using feature extraction, where meaningful data features are automatically constructed by an algorithm. Feature extraction in shallow ML is a manual process that requires domain knowledge of the data that we are learning from.

Neural networks and deep learning concepts leverage statistical techniques and signal processing techniques – which include processing and transformations which are nonlinear. Since nonlinear functions are generally not attributed by a straight line, the relationship between the dependent and independent variables (output and input, respectively) requires more than a slope for the modeling. Functions that are nonlinear include logarithmic terms, polynomial terms, and exponential terms. Nonlinear transformations are often adopted to model several phenomena in the human environment. The same applies to ML and AI solutions as it concerns transformations between the input and output layers.[13]

Large numbers of input features in the data can cause poor performance of DL algorithms. Dimensionality reduction reduces the number of input features using methods like feature selection, linear algebra methods, projection methods, and autoencoders. The benefits of dimensionality reduction are:

- Simplification
- Computational reduction
- Memory power reduction

Following are the examples of deep learning algorithms:

- Convolutional neural networks (CNN)
- Recurrent neural networks (RNN)
- Recursive neural networks (RCNN)
- Deep belief networks (DBN)
- Convolutional deep belief networks (CDBN)
- Feed-forward neural networks (FNN)
- Self-organizing maps (SOM)
- Multi-layer perceptron (MLP)
- Deep Boltzmann machines (DBM)
- Stacked de-noising auto-encoders (SDAE)
- Gated Recurrent Unit (GRU)

Before DL can be leveraged for proffering solutions to problems, some factors must be considered, including:

- Selection of algorithms
- Implementation of algorithms
- Performance assessment of algorithms

Computer Vision

It is an interdisciplinary field that deals with empowering computers to deal with images and videos. More generally, it seeks to automate visual tasks that humans can do.

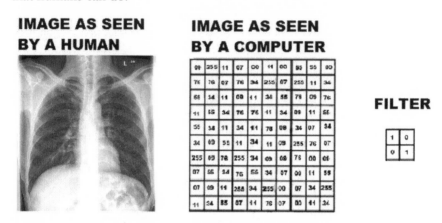

Figure 4-20: Chest radiograph image as seen by a human and a computer, and an example of a filter (small matrix).

The discovery of convolutional neural networks, popularly known as CNNs by Yann LeCun in 1988, revolutionized this field. CNN is a unique framework of the artificial neural network. CNN was designed to function as the human visual cortex, which is responsible for vision. Among the most popular uses of CNN is image identification or classification. For instance, Facebook makes use of CNNs for its auto-tagging feature. Amazon uses CNNs to create product recommendations, while Google uses them to search the photos of its users. Image classification will play an important role in all medical specialties, particularly in the diagnosis of medical images in radiology, pathology, dermatology, orthopedics, ophthalmology, and more.

Computers are able to detect, classify, and locate objects in images and videos using CNNs along with some additional layers of pooling and dense layers. Together they are able to understand the contents in images and videos. Let us learn more about the use of CNNs for the classification (differentiation) of images. The major function that image classification does is to accept the input image and then define the group/type it belongs to. People learn this skill from birth, and as a result, they can conveniently identify pictures of animals and daily use objects. A trained doctor can easily identify the image to be a chest X-ray. However, what the computer sees is quite different.

A computer can never see an image as a person does. Instead, it sees an array of pixels [See Figure 4-20]. For instance, if the size of an image is 300 x 300 pixels, in this situation, the array size will become 300 x 300 x 3. 300 stands for the width, the other 300 stands for the height, while 3 is the value of RGB (Red, Green, and Blue) channels. The value assigned by a computer ranges from 0 to 255 to every one of these specific numbers. This value defines the intensity of a pixel at a particular point.[14,15]

If the computer wants to find a solution to this challenge, it will, first of all, search for the low-level features. According to human understanding, such features, for instance, are either the shoulder bones, ribs, or air-filled lungs. However, for a computer, the edges, curvatures, or boundaries are low-level features. Also, with the help of groups of convolutional layers (forming the whole network), the computer can see more of the high-level features (shoulder bones, ribs, heart, or the air-filled lungs).[14,15]

To explain in detail, the image passes via a series of convolutional, nonlinear, pooling, and fully connected layers. Then it produces the output [see Figures 4-20 and 4-21].

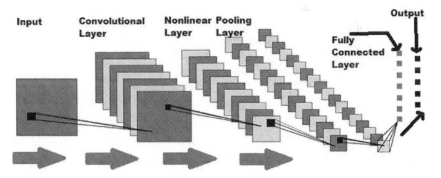

Figure 4-21. Image data passes through various layers of a neural network

The convolutional layer always comes first. The matrix of pixel values (the image) is added to it. Just imagine that the input matrix reading starts from the top left of the image. The software chooses a small matrix there, which is known as a filter (or a core or a neuron). Then this filter creates a convolution, i.e., it moves along the input image. The function of the filter is the multiplication of its values by the original values of the pixel. All of the multiplications are then added up to obtain a single number. The filter starts reading the image from its top left corner and gradually moves further right by a unit after carrying out the multiplication operation. When it reaches the right edge of the image and completes the multiplication operation there, it moves to the left side one row below and continues with the process. After moving the filter through every position on the image, it now obtains a matrix that is smaller than the input matrix [see Figure 4-22].

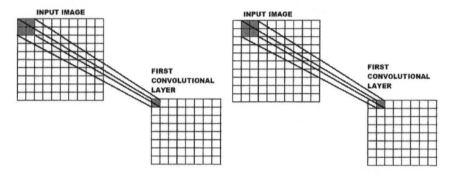

Figure 4-22. The filter starts reading the input image data from its top left corner and gradually moves further right by a unit after carrying out the multiplication operation. The filter moves through every position on the image to obtain a matrix that is smaller than the input matrix

The whole network is required to recognize top-level features in an image, and it consists of several convolutional networks (layers) mixed with nonlinear and pooling layers. When the image passes through one convolutional layer, the output of the first layer becomes the input for the second layer. And this happens with every further convolutional layer. After every convolution operation, a nonlinear layer is included. It contains activation functions that feature nonlinear properties. This property enables a network to be highly intense. After the nonlinear comes the pooling layer. It is concerned with the height and the width of the image and carries out downsampling on the image (decreased image data). This means that if some features (like edges) have already been identified in the previous convolution operation, then a detailed image is no longer needed for further processing, and it is compressed to less detailed pictures. It is vital to include a fully connected layer (dense layers) after completing a series of convolutional, nonlinear, and pooling layers. The function of this layer is to carry data from the convolutional networks.

Computer vision is used for:

- Object Classification

- Object Identification

- Object Verification

- Object Detection

- Object Landmark Detection

- Object Segmentation

- Object Recognition

Outside of just recognition, other methods of analysis include:

- Video motion analysis

- Image segmentation

- Scene reconstruction

- Image restoration

Natural Language Processing (NLP)

NLP is a technology that is aimed at enabling people and computers to communicate with each other on equal footing. It combines knowledge from linguistics with all the latest methods in AI and computer science [see Figure 4-23]. For NLP to function, first, it is important to work on language recognition, i.e., to see if the current model can recognize that language properly. Currently, there are many models available for English, French, German, etc. NLP might not work on regional languages or languages which are less spoken. NLP is viewed as a promising technology within the domain of Human Computer Interface (HCI) to control devices or web applications.[16] The work of chatbots or digital voice assistants was originally based on the principle of NLP. NLP was developed in the 1950s when the scientist Alan Turing wrote and published an article called 'Computing Machinery and Intelligence' in which he presented a method called the 'Turing Test' to measure AI, which is still being used.

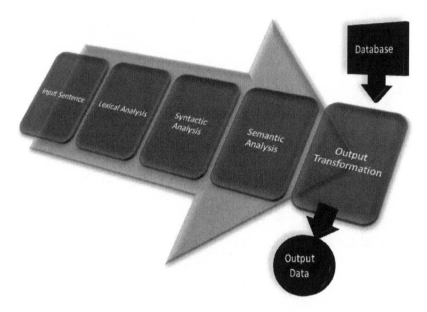

Figure 4-23. A flowchart explaining natural language processing

As early as 1954, researchers had already been able to use a machine to translate sixty sentences into the Russian language. Excited by this breakthrough, several other computer scientists believed that machine translation would soon be possible. However, it was not until the 1980s that the first systems for statistical-based machine translations were further developed. Meanwhile, some other approaches were found that translated information from the 'real' world into the language of computers.[16]

The late 1980s saw another revolutionary breakthrough as ML gained popularity. Along with the ever-increasing computing power of computers, NLP's algorithms were now functional.

Today, NLP-based computer programs can not only use datasets that have been collected manually, but they are also able to analyze text corpora like websites or spoken languages independently. The basis of NLP is the simple concept that any form of language (either spoken or written) should initially be recognized. Nonetheless, language is an incredibly complex system of characters – it is not just a word on its own that is important, but it is the connection that the word has with the other words, phrases, entire sentences, and even facts that is significant as well. While learning from birth is natural for humans, computers have to achieve this using algorithms. Humans are able to access their life experiences, but computers have to access artificially-created experiences.

NLP has various use cases; the most popular uses include:

- Content categorization.

- Topic discovery and modeling.

- Contextual extraction.

- Sentiment analysis.

- Speech-to-text and text-to-speech conversion.

- Document summarization.

- Machine translation.

Choosing the right algorithm

To choose the right algorithm, we need to try out some algorithms which fit our use case and pick the one which performs best on our dataset [see Figure 4-24]. There are no hard and fast rules regarding this, but it's more based on trial and error and experience.

To create a model, one must pass through these phases:

- Construction of the model

- Training the model

- Testing the model

- Evaluation of the model

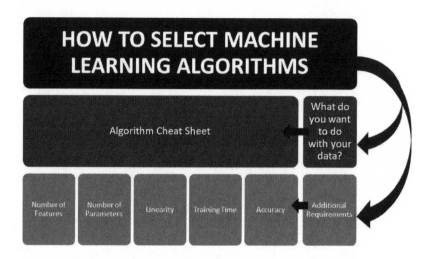

Figure 4-24. Flowchart showing machine learning algorithm selection criteria

Model Creation

Machine learning and deep learning models are usually created in the following manner:

- Selecting a specific kind of algorithm and then defining its parameters and hyperparameters.

- Training the model on labeled data.

- Evaluating the model's performance.

- Using it for prediction.

Model Evaluation

Model evaluation is an essential part of the ML workflow. There's no universal measure that is common to all. Instead, different types of measures are used to evaluate performance, which changes according to the problem being tackled. Some commonly used methods are:

- Accuracy

- Log Loss (Logarithmic Loss)

- Confusion Metrics

- Area Under Curve (AUC)

- F1 Score

- Mean Absolute Error (MAE)

- Mean Squared Error (MSE)

Model Training

Training refers to the process of feeding data to the algorithm to make it learn from the data. Training duration is the time that is taken by the algorithm to learn from the data. It depends on many factors. Simpler models can be trained in a very short duration with a small dataset. In comparison, larger datasets consume a lot of time to learn. The complexity of a model also affects the training time.

Parameters

Parameters are the knobs that can be turned to get different results from the model. The duration of the training and the algorithm's accuracy depends on these parameters. Parameters are learned from data during the training process.

Hyperparameters

Hyperparameters are the adjustable values required for the model, and these are not learned from data.

Determination of optimal hyperparameters for a machine learning model is called tuning. It creates and tests several models having different combinations of settings.[17] The metrics are then compared across all models, and best-performing settings are selected for use.

Although this is a great way to get the best hyperparameter values, the time it takes to train a model exponentially increases with the number of parameters. The benefit is that the presence of numerous parameters usually indicates that an algorithm has more flexibility. Often, it achieves excellent accuracy if one hits the correct combination of parameter settings.[4]

Python libraries for machine learning

Python is 2nd most used programming language in the world. One of the numerous reasons why Python is extremely popular with programmers is that there is a surprisingly huge collection of libraries that users can work with. The following reasons explain why Python enjoys immense popularity:

- Python is relatively easy to learn due to its clear structure and is therefore very suitable for beginners. Its programming syntax is relatively easier to learn and is at a higher level than C, C++, and Java.

- Portability is very important for Python.

- From development to deployment and maintenance, Python helps its developers be more productive.

- Python allows for relatively faster development of new applications with lesser written code.

- Due to the simplicity of Python, many developers have created new machine learning libraries. Python is immensely popular with experts because of this huge collection of libraries.[18]

TensorFlow

It is a free and open-source software library for machine learning and deep learning. It was developed by the Google Brain team, and later it was released as an open-source library. It is available for all major platforms like Windows, macOS, Linux, Android, and iOS.

- TensorFlow provides easy visualization of any part of a diagram, something that is not offered by other libraries.

- TensorFlow can train on CPU (Central Processing Unit), GPU, and TPU (Tensor Processing Unit) as well.

- TensorFlow offers pipelining using which neural networks can be trained on multiple GPUs reducing training time

- Since it was developed by Google, there is a large team of software developers who are constantly working on improvements to make the system more stable and add new features.

TensorFlow is very popular. All libraries created in TensorFlow have been written in either C or C++. Tensorflow mainly supports Python and C++. Some other languages are also being added to it.[19]

During development, first, the Python code is compiled, after which it is executed on the TensorFlow engine using C and C++.

SciKit-Learn

It is also called sklearn. SciKit-Learn is a Python library that is linked to both SciPy and NumPy. It is a free library that supports multiple machine learning algorithms, including ones like SVMs, Random Forests, k-means clustering, etc. It originally started as a Google Summer of Code project. It is written in Python and uses Numpy and SciPy for high-performance mathematical operations.

The SciKit-Learn library contains a variety of algorithms for implementing standard tasks for machine learning and data mining. These include reducing dimensionality, classification, regression, clustering, and model selection.

NumPy

NumPy is one of the most popular libraries for machine learning in Python. It supports large multi-dimensional arrays and matrices and high-level mathematical functions to operate on these arrays. It is an open-source library. It was developed to simplify array operations and increase performance. It is an abbreviated form of Numerical Python.

TensorFlow and other libraries use NumPy internally to perform various operations.

- NumPy is both very interactive and incredibly easy to use.

- NumPy helps make mathematically complex implementations easy.

- It makes it easier for one to code and grasp the concepts.

- NumPy is widely used, so there are many open-source implementations.

The NumPy interface can be used for the expression of images, sound waves, as well as other data in the form of an array of real numbers in the N dimensions.

Keras

It is also an open-source library that is written in Python. It now acts as an interface for the Tensorflow library. Its previous versions also supported various backends like Tensorflow, Theano, R, etc. Its design supports the fast development of models which is used for experimental purpose. It also supports training on GPUs as well as TPUs. Keras models can also be deployed on multiple platforms like web, android, iOS, etc.

Keras is one of the most impressive learning libraries for Python, and it offers a simple mechanism for the representation of neural networks. However, Keras is comparatively slower than other ML libraries because it creates a computational graph through the backend infrastructure and uses it to complete the processes. All the models in Keras are portable, regardless.

- Keras runs smoothly on both the GPU and the CPU.

- Keras practically supports almost all kinds of neural networks, whether they are fully connected, pooled, recurring, embedded, etc. Additionally, different types may be combined to create more complex models.

- The modular structure of Keras makes it incredibly expressive, ideal, and flexible for innovative research.

- Being a completely Python-based framework, Keras simplifies solving the problem and exploring this library.

You might be using applications that use Keras-based models on a daily basis. Apps like Netflix, Yelp, Uber, Zocdoc, Instacart, and Square, among many others, use Keras. It is a popular notion with startups that make use of deep learning technology.

Moreover, it offers a great choice of pre-trained models such as MNIST, VGG, Inception, SqueezeNet, ResNet, etc. Lastly, Keras is preferred by deep learning researchers. It is already used by researchers who work in large scientific organizations, like NASA and CERN.[11]

PyTorch

PyTorch is another popular deep learning framework. It is also a free and open-source library. It also offers a C++ interface along with the main Python interface. Caffe2 was merged into PyTorch in 2018. It feels more native to Python as compared to other frameworks.

The PyTorch library is based on Torch, which is an open-source library that is implemented in C with a wrapper in Lua. PyTorch in Python was officially introduced in 2017. From the time of its foundation, the library has become increasingly popular and has attracted more and more machine learning developers.[17]

- Research and production performance is optimized by leveraging native support for asynchronous execution of collective operations as well as peer-to-peer communications that is accessible through Python and C++.

- PyTorch is not simply an integration of Python into a monolithic C++ framework – it is designed to be deeply integrated into Python to allow for its usage with common packages and libraries like Cython or Numba.

A dynamic community of developers and researchers has created a wide range of both tools and libraries for the expansion of PyTorch, and in doing so, supports the development in the area from computer vision to reinforcement learning.

PyTorch is used mostly for applications like NLP. It was originally developed by Facebook's AI research group. TensorFlow & PyTorch are both competing frameworks. It is attracting a good amount of attention, majorly in the research community.

Light GBM

It stands for Light Gradient Boosting Machine. It was originally developed by Microsoft. It is an open-source framework that also works on distributed machines. It is also compatible with popular languages like Python, R, C++, etc. It uses decision trees. It is designed for high performance.

It aids developers in the creation of new algorithms via newly defined elementary models and, particularly, decision trees. There are special libraries designed to implement this method swiftly and effectively – LightGBM, CatBoost, and XGBoost.[16] All these libraries are 'competitors' but aid in solving a common problem and can also be used in almost similar ways.

- Faster training speed and higher efficiency.

- Lower memory usage.

- Better accuracy.

- Support of parallel and GPU learning.

- Capable of handling large-scale data.

This library offers implementation of gradient boosting that is optimized, scalable, and rapid, making it highly popular with the developers of ML.

Eli5

It is a python library that is used for debugging ML and DL code. It also explains predictions made by models. It provides support for numerous libraries like scikit-learn, Keras, XGBoost, LightGBM, etc.

It is a combination of visualization and debugging for machine learning models, tracking steps of the algorithm. Most machine learning and deep learning models are also called black boxes as we don't know what's happening inside them and how they are learning it. It helps in model interpretation for those who don't understand the terminologies related to ML and DL.

In scikit-learn, it allows explaining weights and predictions of classifiers and regressors. It can print decision trees as text and many more.

SciPy

It is also referred to as Scientific Python. SciPy is an environment containing open-source libraries that are particularly helpful in Science, Mathematics, and Engineering. Some of its core packages are (also called SciPy stack):

- NumPy

- SciPy library

- Matplotlib

- IPython

- SymPy

- Pandas

SciPy is used in scientific computing, along with NumPy. SciPy makes use of NumPy as the integral data structure, and it incorporates the modules for various commonly used tasks in scientific programming like integration (calculus), linear algebra, common solving of differential equations, and signal processing.[17]

Theano

Theano is a python-based library and optimizing compiler for matrix-related computation of multidimensional arrays. It is built on top of NumPy. It may also be used in parallel or distributed environments that are similar to TensorFlow.[17]

- It is possible to make use of whole arrays of NumPy in functions that are Theano-compiled.

- Transparent usage of GPUs.

- Data-intensive calculations can be carried out a lot faster.

- Theano performs the derivation for functions that have either one or more inputs.

- Theano is very stable even for complex calculations

- Includes tools for diagnosing bugs

Theano's actual syntax is symbolic and can be difficult for beginners. Expressions are particularly defined in an abstract manner, compiled, and used later for the actual calculation.[18]

Theano was originally designed specifically for calculations that are needed for large neural network algorithms like the ones that are used in deep learning. Developed in 2007, Theano was one of the first libraries of its kind, due to which it is seen as the industry standard for deep learning and development. Additionally, it is utilized in several neural network projects nowadays, and its popularity is on the rise.

Pandas

It is a very powerful library that is built using Python. It is used for data analysis and data manipulation.

Pandas comes with the provision of high-level data structures and an assortment of analysis tools. One of its best features is its ability to translate complex data operations through just one or two commands. Pandas even has several integrated methods for the grouping, combining, and filtering of data, including time-series functionality. Supporting processes like iteration, re-indexing, sorting, aggregation, visualization, and chaining is one of the highlights of the library.

Pandas data frames can handle large amounts of data and can perform manipulations like finding missing values, organizing data in specific formats like in date and time. It also enables the reading and writing of data from different file types and doing operations on them. It also makes file format conversion very easy. It is a very important library in Data Science and Data Analytics.

Matplotlib

- It is a very popular library that is used to create visualizations and graphs in Python. It is used to plot interactive graphs and figures in 2-D and 3-D. In machine learning and deep learning, data visualization plays an important role. Using matplotlib, we can easily create plots describing various properties of data, which helps us in formulating better models. Graphs are also helpful in comparing the performance of the model with time and to other models as well.

References/Further Reading

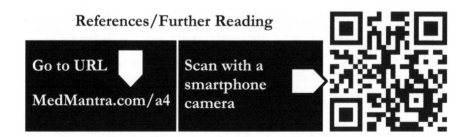

Go to URL
MedMantra.com/a4

Scan with a smartphone camera

CHAPTER FIVE

THE AI BLACK BOX ISSUE AND EXPLAINABLE AI

AI is now an essential component of our lives. Practically, it is employed in almost every field. AI is involved in lots of decision-making. AI products are also marketed as safer alternatives because they lack chances of human error. In specific domains like healthcare, predicting diseases such as cancer and the development of new and better medicines is done using deep learning (DL). It is the human tendency to find the logic behind a decision that makes the decision more trustworthy. Most DL-generated results lack any logical explanation. Besides, most of us don't understand the technicalities related to AI. Sometimes, decisions are hard to trust; this is where the actual problem starts. Earlier, people were satisfied with the results they were getting from the implementation of AI; now, they want to know the reasoning behind the formation of results. Therefore, Explainable AI (XAI) is the next big thing.

The black box issue

Essentially, the black box issue stands tall because the workings of DL algorithms are difficult to understand. We feed DL models with vast amounts of training data so that they learn from it. After that, we input data at one end, and on the other side, we get the predicted output. But what happens in between remains a mystery. These models do not give details about how they arrived at any decision. These decisions are very opaque.[1] Conventional ML algorithms are transparent (white box); however, modern DL algorithms are opaque (black box).

Thus, it gets quite hard for professionals in the field to explain how these models do it, usually when presenting these ideas or results to different stakeholders or investors or the common public. No doubt, the DL models employ mathematical functions and values, which is not a mystery or magic. However, it is a bit harder to explain how they work to people who lack related technical know-how.

Why it is important

On the whole, people believe that they have the right to know how and why a particular decision was made. This is highly important in terms of the healthcare sector because patients want to know the answer to the question of how and why they're supposed to believe this information. More than that, the doctors wish to understand the reasoning behind the AI's decision.

The hidden problems

AI algorithms learn on their own based solely on the training data. This data may contain hidden biases and human prejudices. These hidden traits in data do affect decisions dramatically. Algorithms lack morale, which is a vital part of any human decision.

AI often predicts unfair or wrong decisions due to these hidden features of data. This has been observed several times. Its most prominent example is the *COMPAS* case.[2] **COMPAS**, an acronym for Correctional Offender Management Profiling for Alternative Sanctions, is assistive AI-based software that helped judges decide whether to detain a defendant before trials. Its creators ignored the biases contained in the training data. Its predictions in the case of black defendants failed utterly. The software labeled black defendants as being twice riskier than their white counterparts. Many US state jurisdiction authorities used it. The case showed that data must be carefully assessed and then fed into the model.

This is problematic not only for lack of transparency but also for the correctness of the decision. AI has a significant impact on various people's lives. Such biases can have disastrous effects in real life. They must be appropriately addressed, especially with the implementation of AI in the healthcare sector.

Why explainable AI?

If AI could explain the produced answer, this would add to its credibility. It will also help us tackle all the biases and prejudices hidden in the training data. Using XAI, one can know what went wrong. Then, software engineers can work that out, ultimately boosting the performance. We will also get insights into the workings of these systems.

From multiple perspectives, XAI seems promising.

There can be two approaches for XAI:

- Explanation by Design,

- And Black Box Explanation.

In the former, a model can be trained to produce an explanation along with the decision. The latter approach suggests developing models that can explain the results from a black box model perspective. Both methods are useful in their approaches.

Black box issues in healthcare

Trust is a massive factor in medical treatment. Unless we are sure of a particular decision or treatment, we cannot risk it. Believing the prediction or recommendation by AI algorithms without knowing why and how is hard. Lack of transparency in healthcare can have serious consequences. Healthcare professionals are very much answerable for their decisions legally as well; they cannot merely say that AI recommended it unless they know the reason behind it.

One such study was conducted by Riccardo Moitto and colleagues[3]; it was called Deep Patient on Electronic Health Records (EHRs). It aimed to predict the health status of its patients and help prevent further disease or disability. According to the study, it was quite successful in providing the right diagnosis to patients. While it was helpful to a great extent, it also proved to be a black box. It was able to predict the onset of mental disorders in patients. There was no clear explanation of how these predictions were made, but they proved to be true over time, leading to baffled doctors.

While AI is significantly helping in the healthcare sector, the creation of the black box leaves professionals utterly confused. Thus, there is a focus on XAI and creating more transparent algorithms for people to understand and work with.

Layer-wise Relevance Propagation (LRP)

This is a very appropriate method in explainable AI. It can be easily applied to pre-trained models. LRP uses layer-wise weights and activations to calculate their contribution to the overall prediction. Using it, we can inspect what made a model predict this output. LRP can be used on Convolutional Neural Networks (CNNs), Long Short-Term Memory cells (LSTMs), and other deep learning algorithms.

It can be easily implemented in most programming languages.

Other useful techniques

Several machine learning algorithms like decision trees and Bayesian networks are easy to interpret. They can be visualized easily, and we can explain their predictions. We can see what properties were used as a decisive factor and how much they affected the predictions.

Some XAI frameworks

What-if Tool:

This is made by the TensorFlow team. It is an interactive visual interface designed to visualize datasets[4] and better understand the TensorFlow model output.

DeepLift:

This assigns contribution scores to each neuron involved in the model, which is used for prediction. It considers positive and negative contributions differently and gives them scores accordingly. It can also reveal dependencies that other approaches might not detect.

Activation Atlases:

This is developed by the combined efforts of Google and OpenAI. It aims to visualize how neural networks interact with each other. It is developed to visualize the inner workings of CNNs so that humans can easily understand them.

Future of XAI

Explainable AI is a field of active research. New algorithms are being worked out to solve the black box AI problems. Model transparency and explanation are very much needed in this digital society.

References/Further Reading

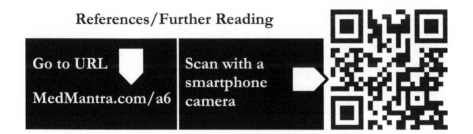

Go to URL

MedMantra.com/a6

Scan with a smartphone camera

CHAPTER SIX

THE FUTURE OF AI IN HEALTHCARE WITH FEDERATED LEARNING

Machine learning (ML) is constantly evolving. One of the latest developments is federated learning (FL), which was introduced in 2017 by Google AI researchers.[1,2] Here is a complete guide to what federated learning is and the future of AI in healthcare with federated learning.

The Basics of Federated Learning

In conventional methods of ML, a data pipeline utilizes a central data server, which pools data from local data sources, and the local training nodes acquire data from this server to train ML models locally [see Figure 6-1 A]. The problem with this method is that the data must be transferred from the central server to the local training nodes. For that reason, the ML model is limited in its ability to learn in real-time.

There are two types of FL workflows: the aggregation server FL workflow and the peer-to-peer FL workflow.[3] In the aggregation server FL workflow, the most current ML model is downloaded and an updated model is computed in the local training nodes/computers using local data. These updated models are sent from the training nodes to the central (aggregation) server, where they are aggregated [see Figure 6-1 B]. Aggregation means that an improved global and consolidated model is computed and sent back to the local training nodes. In the peer-to-peer FL workflow, there is no central aggregation server and the aggregation is performed by each local training node (a peer). Initially, all local training nodes are synchronized so that they have the same, most current ML model [see Figure 6-1 C]. An updated model is computed by the local training nodes using local data. These updated models are exchanged by the participating nodes such that each node has all the updated models. Each node then aggregates these updated models so that each one has the same updated global model.

Because of FL, the ML algorithms gain experience from a wide range of data sets in different locations. In short, it allows many organizations to collaborate without sharing their sensitive data.

FL decentralizes the process of machine learning, as it removes the need for pooling data into a single location (the central server). Only the characteristics of the model are transferred, such as gradients, parameters, etc. The model is trained at different locations in different iterations. The process repeats for several iterations until a high-quality model is developed [see Figures 6-1 B and 6-1 C].

Here are the five most important benefits of FL[4,5]:

- Patient data privacy is maintained.

- The models are smarter – FL-trained models are superior and have incredible performance levels compared to models that see data from only one institute.

- It allows for better clinical decision-making. Clinicians can use their own expertise in conjunction with knowledge from other healthcare institutions to diagnose and treat diseases. Patients in remote areas can also benefit from such a model, as they have access to better care.

- Predictions are made locally, so latency is lowered.

- Once the FL model is successfully implemented in healthcare centers, it allows for unbiased decision-making without data privacy and governance concerns.

- When the FL model is used, it is much easier to become a data donor. This is because patients know that their data will remain safe and the accessibility can be revoked at any time

Now that you know the basics of FL, let's move onto understanding the future of this AI model in healthcare.

FL and Data Privacy Issues

The problem with conventional methods of ML is that they pose a risk to patient data privacy in the healthcare industry. Such a risk hinders the progress of AI in the life sciences and healthcare. However, FL can help in dealing with data privacy issues.

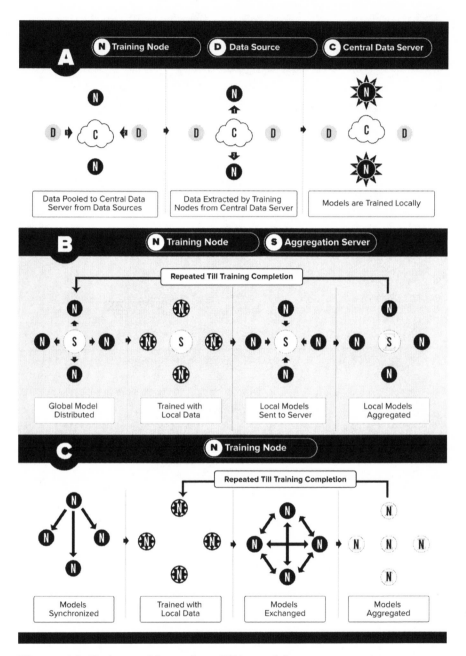

Figure 6-1. Federated Learning (FL) workflows

Previously, many researchers proved that even anonymized health datasets can be used to re-identify patients.[6] Other research has shown that MRI or CT data can help reconstruct the faces of the patients.[7,8] Of course, because of these possibilities, there are concerns with patient data privacy.

Many have wondered if one must compromise to benefit from AI models in healthcare. However, FL has changed the game entirely, as the ML algorithms in this model are trained locally. This means the patients' data is not shared outside the privacy of the hospital/institution. The model has privacy-preserving techniques, which include data being stored locally and neither leaked to a third party nor sent to the cloud/central server. Decision-making becomes better due to these privacy-preserving techniques. Also, real-time predictions are made possible because the process happens on the local device. Such a model has long been needed in the healthcare industry.

FL follows all compliance and consent requirements and regulations. These include the European Union's General Data Protection Regulation, HIPAA, and many others. Compliance is achieved by ensuring that all data remains within the network of the healthcare organization.

How FL Can Help Healthcare CIOs

CIOs (Chief Information Officers) are responsible for leading the IT (Information Technology) departments of healthcare organizations. Here are some of the key tasks they carry out:

- Assessing current and future technology needs

- Devising strategic initiatives to advance data-driven innovation

- Devising strategic initiatives to diversify revenue streams

- Managing and improving the technology spend of the healthcare organization

- Leveraging the organization's data for research and revenue purposes

The problem with achieving some of these aims is that a lack of resources prevents existing data from being made available for collaboration or used effectively. Leveraging data cost-effectively and efficiently is one of the most essential goals right now in the healthcare industry.

That is why CIOs should work toward unlocking the value of the existing data instead of focusing on gathering more data. They should seek out FL models that are capable of ensuring data security and privacy. Such security should be not only in the data but also in the code utilized to write the FL algorithms.

If CIOs implement such an FL system, they can foster collaborative data, diversify revenue streams, and achieve data-driven innovation for their healthcare organizations. Here are many other ways an FL system can help CIOs[9]:

1. *Accessibility and Security*

All data collected by the FL model is kept locally, which improves the physical data transfer speeds and reduces the risk of a data leak. People authorized to access the data can do so effectively and securely from any location. That is why the CIOs have more accessibility and everyone in the organization benefits from higher security.

2. *Compliance and Privacy*

Any FL model is created in compliance with various rules, regulations, and standards. These ensure that the data stay in the healthcare organization and are protected. Thus, using an FL model ensures compliance and privacy. The CIOs can then focus on other aspects of improving the healthcare organization.

3. *De-Risked Correlation*

One of the most important things in clinical research is the ability to correlate with various data sets. This is because local data sets are small and can be biased. Also, the correlating data can become de-anonymized and linked.

FL can encourage more secure data correlation. It can offer differential privacy, which allows for data sharing by describing patterns of groups within the data sets. All this can be done by withholding information about individuals and protecting patient privacy.

4. *Integration*

Healthcare data is vast and expansive. Patients have a long history of healthcare, and this data needs to be consolidated and integrated. Previous ML models did not achieve this aim well.

However, with FL, the existing healthcare databases can be integrated and organized. The structuring of data becomes easier, actionable, and searchable. All authorized persons can access integrated data to better understand the patients' medical history.

The FL model can help CIOs achieve these four aims so that their organizations can progress in terms of technology and revenue. After all, every healthcare organization needs to work towards achieving these goals to provide a better experience for their patients.

FL Applications That Are Being Used Today

Keep in mind that the FL model is relatively new as compared to the other ML models. It still has a long way to go before it can prove its validity in a regulated and productive environment. As of now, a few healthcare technology providers are rolling out and making use of this technology.

For example, the ML startup Owkin has come up with a new FL platform known as *Owkin Connect*.[10] The platform gives data owners the capabilities to track their data usage and define their data authorizations. A ledger keeps track of the data being used by the model for training and how it contributes to the parameters of the model.

On the other hand, the ACR Data Science Institute is piloting a new FL framework for medical devices, known as *NVIDIA Clara FL*.[11] It is a toolkit that democratizes AI by providing radiologists with the capabilities to develop algorithms using the patient data at their healthcare organizations. There is still a long way to go before FL becomes as common as the previous ML models.

Of course, many companies are working on the technology and we will soon see many applications being rolled out that will help healthcare organizations. The technology will put the patient or user in charge of coordinating their health data. More effective models will be built using the FL architecture. That is why it is likely the future of AI in healthcare.

Challenges With FL

All AI models come with a few sets of challenges that must be overcome. One of the main challenges of the FL models is communication. Because the FL models are trained using data generated by local devices, efficient communication must be developed.

That is because if there are too many communication rounds, it will require more time, effort, and resources. Besides that, small model updates will have to be sent as part of training instead of sending the entire dataset altogether. Developing efficient communication methods is key to building a successful FL framework.

Another challenge with FL models is the anticipation of low levels of device participation. That means only a handful of devices will be active at once. Few devices will be able to tolerate variability in the hardware that affects the communication, computational, and storage capabilities of each device in the network.

Lastly, communicating model updates during the training phase of the model has a chance of revealing sensitive information. Such information can be leaked to either the central server in the network or a third party. These challenges must be overcome for the model to be a success in the healthcare industry.

Of course, this AI model is relatively new, and research to test it is still being carried out. Once we know more about this model, researchers can devise ways to overcome these challenges for a better experience.

The Future of Digital Health With FL

Many studies and much research have been done on FL. Recent studies have shown that the models trained by FL can help achieve performance levels that are superior to older models that see data from only one institute.

There is high potential once the FL model is successfully implemented. It can lead to unbiased decisions, better patient privacy and data governance, and an accurate reflection of the physiology of each individual.[3] The FL model shows a lot of promise in overcoming the limitations of models that require centralized data from a single pool.

That is why it is said that the future of digital health lies with FL. It promises one essential thing that has been missing from previous ML models: patient privacy and data governance. Each data controller in the FL model:

- Defines its governance process

- Defines its associated privacy policies

- Controls data access

- Has the capability to revoke data access

All these aims can be met in the validation and training phases. That is why FL has the potential to create many new opportunities in the healthcare industry. It can enable much-needed research on rare diseases and allow large-scale institutional validation inside a healthcare organization.

The FL model can also scale naturally. It can grow global data sets without disproportionately increasing data storage requirements. That is why it can help healthcare organizations naturally scale in the long run as well.

FL now provides an opportunity to capture higher data variability and analyze patients across different demographics. For example, in the context of EHR (electronic health records), FL can find and represent clinically similar patients.[12] Besides that, it can make predictions of hospitalizations based on ICU stay time[13], cardiac events[14], and mortality.

The FL model has the power to create a direct clinical impact. For example, the *HealthChain* project aims to deploy an FL framework in France across four hospitals.[15] The framework will generate common models that make predictions of treatment response for melanoma and breast cancer patients.

The framework will help oncologists determine what course of treatment to take for their patients. It will demonstrate the response based on dermoscopy images and histology slides. That is just one of the examples of how FL is already affecting digital health.

Another promising example is that of *FeTS (Federated Tumour Segmentation)*.[16] This is an international federation consisting of thirty healthcare institutions using an open-source FL framework. This framework aims to improve tumor boundary detection from various myeloma patients.

However, the application of the FL framework in digital health is not just on treatment response or disease detection. Instead, the application extends to industrial translation and research as well. That is because FL allows for collaborative research.

One of the biggest initiatives of the FL framework for this purpose is the *Melloddy* project, which aims to deploy multi-task FL across data sets of ten pharmaceutical companies.[17] The pharmaceutical partners aim to optimize the drug discovery process by training a common predictive model. The model will infer how chemical compounds bind to proteins. The partners will be able to achieve the aims of this model without revealing their data.

Many clinicians have already improved diagnostic tools for imaging analysis through the use of FL models. Additionally, pharma companies are reducing their costs and saving their time to market with accelerated and collaborative drug discovery. In the future, the FL model has the potential to increase the robustness and accuracy of healthcare AI tools while improving the outcome for patients and decreasing costs.

In the coming decades, the FL model will improve medical care, diagnosis, treatment response, disease detection, and much more. We will just have to wait and see how it all happens.

Conclusion

That was your complete guide to the FL models being used across healthcare industries. It is the most promising AI model we have right now. However, it is still in its initial phase; more research is necessary to completely understand its potential.

It is showing much promise in the field of healthcare and we can't wait to see more companies coming up with the latest FL technology. It is the future of healthcare and might soon take over the industry.

References/Further Reading

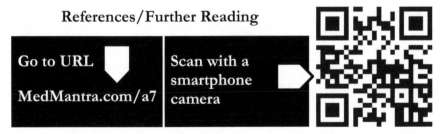

Go to URL
MedMantra.com/a7

Scan with a smartphone camera

CHAPTER SEVEN

MYTHS ABOUT AI APPLICATIONS IN HEALTHCARE

It takes at least a decade of hard work and experience to become a doctor, but still, they misdiagnose cases. Even the best of doctors make mistakes, and medical errors are now the third most leading cause of death in the US.[1] It's neither the doctor's fault nor is the deficiency in training; human nature is liable to make mistakes, and such mistakes in hospital settings might cost one his/her life.

This is where artificial intelligence or AI comes to the rescue. The ability of AI-enabled systems to work at super-human speed tirelessly has attracted billions of dollars of investment in the healthcare industry. Until recently, the healthcare industry has had little to no automation—and lacked predictive analytics—and complex protocols to reach a diagnosis. While AI models also need to be trained on a given set of data, just like doctors, they're far better at handling multiple variables at a time, providing logical reasoning and ceaseless analytics that is uninfluenced by sleep, tiredness, or long duty hours. This, in contrast, can provide a low-cost, highly efficient alternative to traditional health care.

As of now, the application of AI is best seen in diagnostic imaging and finding out specific patterns on microscopic slides in pathology. It can point out subtle changes that would otherwise be missed by a doctor, and that, too, in the blink of an eye. As a result of this, many healthcare organizations are attempting to take into account the most revolutionary uses of AI, such as automated diagnostics, MRI/CT/X-ray imaging analysis, histopathological identification of tumors, differentials of dermatology, and automated robotic surgery.

The learning of human-to-human interaction with robots can eventually train the AI model to perform optimally in hospital settings. The implementation of this process can help automate various processes, including referrals to specialists based on a diagnosis, issuing a warning for medicine allergies, automated treatment plans, and claims processing.

AI can help hospital management achieve 'Optimal Operational Performance' and ensure that facilities and equipment are always in use and never scarce, the right number and type of staff are present, and appropriate medical supplies are in hand. AI can also aid in analyzing data from many sources and compile them to increase the quality of health care while keeping the costs low

Myths about AI

Although the implications of AI in health care are vast, certain myths need to be busted before we continue the journey to the era of automated diagnostics.

Myth number 1: AI will replace doctors

Visiting a doctor is expensive! And the added burden of hospital charges and diagnostic costs makes sure that you're just one illness away from bankruptcy. AI, on the other hand, follows the 'zero marginal cost' trend, meaning that the first copy of the software is expensive, and the rest of them are just free. This can eventually make health care affordable and accessible throughout the globe, at least in theory.

Bots have been replacing human jobs since the rise of technological marvels. One report says that almost half of the jobs people are doing right now can be automated by augmenting currently available technologies. Between now and 2030, 400 million persons are estimated to lose their jobs to automation.[2] The AI has already replaced jobs that require repetitive tasks such as those of cashiers, secretaries, travel agencies, video stores, and many others. Here's a breakdown of the job routines in a healthcare setting:

Repetitive	Routine	Optimizing	Complex	Creative
Pharmacology	Hematology	Radiology	Medicine	Interventional Radiology
Medical Reporting	Histopathology	Research Analytics	Surgery	Plastic Surgery

AI is to completely replace the repetitive and routine jobs in coming years, such as those of histopathologists and hematologists. These jobs require a specific pattern recognition or image analysis to reach a diagnosis, and an AI model cannot only outperform but can also notice subtle changes that would otherwise be ignored by a human eye. But an AI-powered system will take more than a decade to autonomously perform more complex procedures and highly skilled jobs. Even with that level of tech development, AI can only perform in a specific niche, and General Artificial Intelligence is still a way off.

Expert doctors working with intelligent software to augment decision-making will perform significantly better than either of them alone. AI algorithms are currently being employed to diagnose minor medical conditions that general practitioners look into and, if proven accurate, can potentially assist the clinical accuracy of doctors.

But what's keeping AI from knocking down doctors on their own turf is the dependency of algorithms on data presets. Machine learning (ML), a branch of AI, requires a lot of data to be fed into the system for an algorithm to analyze and create a logical outcome. This data includes patients' electronic health records (EHR), radiological imaging, blood test values, and so much more. The unavailability of this huge number of processed medical data is the biggest hurdle to AI development.

No two patients are alike. There is even a difference in the anatomical landmarks and disease progression in different people. Although AI can take a 'guess' of possible differentials, it cannot precisely diagnose a case that has never been fed into it, requiring a human expert to tackle such cases.

Training the algorithms is an arduous process. It requires close interaction between the clinicians and the developers to make sure medically authentic data is fed into the training models. While the medical research data doubles every two years, it's hard to imagine an AI system is able to cope up with new trends without a doctor chewing up data variables for it. These tools can get better over time as they learn, which enables them to evolve with new medical research.

AI can, however, augment safe medical practice by helping doctors reach an accurate diagnosis promptly so a timely intervention can be done to save precious lives. AI will be a tech that assists doctors, not substitutes them. It will aid physicians to get more knowledge about the patient's ailment to make an accurate diagnosis and better-informed decisions, enabling the physician to spend more time winning the patient's trust and making emotional bonds. Just as a stethoscope augments a doctor in making a clinical diagnosis, AI is the latest tool that will further enhance the quality of health care.

In a nutshell, doctors will continue to do jobs that require creativity, decision-making skills, and human interaction. Characteristics like sympathy, judgment, creativity, compassion, and analytical reasoning are lacking in bots, so in the areas where human empathy is fundamental, AI-powered robots won't be a replacement. The aforementioned AI tools will continue to automate small repetitive tasks performed by doctors and allow them to focus on the doctor-patient relationship and patient-centered care.

Myth number 2: AI models are biased

What is bias? Bias in medical practice can influence a doctor's diagnostic accuracy and can lead to errors in clinical management. A number of biases can limit rationality and logical reasoning, which a doctor gathers and uses as evidence in making diagnoses. These biases are not limited to the medical field but, rather, are illustrations of suboptimal reasoning people are liable to.

The AI model can be biased if the data it's learning from is biased. This biased AI model can be potentially more harmful because of its vast scale of operation versus a couple of patients a doctor is checking. The art of medical diagnosis is so intricate that a biased AI system can go unnoticed for a long time. There are many subtle ways in which a model can go wrong and pick-up bias that is harmful. Therefore, more fundamental research needs to be done on data used in machine learning to avoid a catastrophe.

Fortunately, a biased AI-model is easy to fix, with correct logical data and retraining the machine algorithms. This continues to be an ongoing topic of research to identify ways of detecting and correcting biases and unreliable data sources.

Myth number 3: AI is too risky to use in healthcare

The scope of AI implementations in health care is tremendous—from diagnostics to research data collection to augmented surgeries—for revolutionizing the delivery of healthcare in the modern era. The AI implementation in clinical settings poses a greater risk to the healthcare facility. The stakes of getting the right diagnosis are much higher in this field.

The diagnostic accuracy of AI far exceeds that of top board-certified doctors. So, the risk of AI misdiagnosing a case is at least less than what we have in specialist care institutions. AI is only as good as the data upon which the model is trained, so the success of the AI model is not based much on algorithms but on the data provided to it.

In a head-to-head competition with senior radiologists in China, The BioMind AI system developed at the Beijing Tiantan Hospital made correct diagnoses in 87% of cases in about 15 minutes, while a team of 15 senior professors achieved an accuracy of only 66% in 225 total cases.[3]

Babylon developed an AI-powered app to help diagnose minor ailments or refer to a nearby healthcare facility if symptoms point to a serious condition.

"Babylon's latest artificial intelligence capabilities show that it is possible for anyone, irrespective of their geography, wealth, or circumstances, to have free access to health advice that is on par with top-rated practicing clinicians."

Dr. Parsa – Founder, Babylon

The Royal College of General Practitioners (RCGP) conducts an examination to grant practicing licenses to passing students. The company made its AI take the exam for MRCGP, in which it scored 81%, whereas the passing score is 72%.[4]

So, the advancements in AI can significantly improve the healthcare industry, promising improved patient care and more accurate diagnosis while slightly increasing the associated risks.

Myth number 4: Robotic Process Automation (RPA) will fix data problems

The biggest challenge in the healthcare industry is the sorting of data received from various sources. The new patient forms, medical prescriptions, handwritten notes, medical claims forms, and radiographs all exemplify the challenges of managing disorganized data and implementing its use in research and analytics. There's a misconception that AI will correct the data flow with its 'magic wand.'

AI developers and data scientists need organized, complete, and accurate data—not to mention metadata—to train AI algorithms on how to identify a red flag and return useful results only. Such data is not yet available, and even AI can't solve it.

There is a dire need for smart input software that can collect and organize data from different sources into one place, which enables record stratification and data extraction. This structured data combined with RPA can enable healthcare organizations to deliver data for machine learning. This organization of data can be achieved in the following ways:

- The implementation of one data entry point into the healthcare system. For example, instead of manually inputting data by asking patients every time, the data is automatically populated into the system with identity codes.

- The extraction of metadata from patient forms, ensuring that the concerned information filled out in the form is thoroughly validated and processed by Electronic Health Records (EHR) system.

- The incorporation of unstructured content such as X-ray and prescription information included within relevant forms for processing.

Myth number 5: AI means the end of privacy

There's an argument that AI can be worse than humans when it comes to privacy and security. Unauthorized access to databases containing critical health information can be more damaging than any other data breach in this modern era.

Artificial intelligence exposes us to a wide range of challenges concerning data security and privacy, along with the fact that AI models need massive amounts of structured data for training.

Although machine learning models are trained on anonymous data, some people are still concerned about their personal illnesses being revealed to others who have access to the system. In a study[5], around 90% of data experts said that patients should be concerned about their data being potentially misused when given to healthcare organizations for analytics.

For the coming years, AI development will depend on its access to even bigger and populated medical and healthcare datasets. The tools we have used up until now to protect people's privacy and identification while making the data available for research and analytics cannot be used to secure datasets used for AI development. To make the data available while maintaining privacy, there is a need for the development of modern privacy-enhancing technologies (PET). This will ensure privacy protection in the working environment of AI.

Conclusion

The potential benefits of AI implementation outweigh the risks associated with bringing automation to the medical field. While artificially intelligent robots are not yet there to replace doctors, they can augment doctors' jobs in the healthcare delivery system by taking up repetitive tasks such as analyzing tests, x-rays, MRI and CT scans, data entry, and loads of other tedious tasks. The preliminary progress is promising, but the data privacy and non-availability of massive structured data are stumbling blocks in AI development. In the upcoming years, AI models will get more mature to bring a revolution in the way we diagnose and treat ailments.

"AI is serendipity; it is here to liberate us from monotonous jobs and make us more human."

References/Further Reading

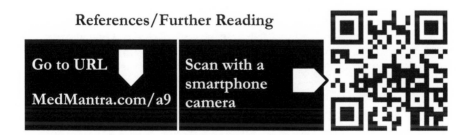

Go to URL	Scan with a smartphone camera
MedMantra.com/a9	

CHAPTER EIGHT

ETHICAL QUESTIONS FOR ARTIFICIAL INTELLIGENCE IN HEALTHCARE

Artificial Intelligence (AI) has long been a point of interest in a number of fields, including medical research and healthcare. With AI seeing rapid advancements throughout the world, there are ethical questions being raised as well. Recently, the Nuffield Council of Bioethics examined the present and possible applications of artificial intelligence in healthcare. The briefing note released in May 2018 by the organization not only looked at how AI can make healthcare more efficient and accessible, it focused on serious ethical questions as well.

The present use of AI in the medical sphere has typically been for disease detection, chronic condition management, healthcare delivery, and discovery of new pharmaceuticals, but AI is being trialed in other components as well. Thus, an examination of ethics is necessary. The Nuffield Council on Bioethics believes that AI "has the potential to help address important health challenges," but AI has limitations that can create some mistrust and discontent, especially regarding privacy and human characteristics.

Some of the ethical questions raised in the briefing note are:

- What is the possibility of AI making errors?

- Who is responsible when the AI system makes the wrong decision?

- What is the potential of AI being used with malicious intent?

- How will AI change the skill requirements of medical professionals? Will less experienced and skilled professionals be able to handle the demands of their job if AI fails?

- How will AI affect a patient's sense of dignity? Further, will AI create social isolation in specific cases?

- What security measures will be used to protect individual privacy and other sensitive data?

Additionally, the briefing note goes into detail about the potential of AI developing issues that cannot be identified or fixed because of the complex nature of artificial intelligence itself. Should such complicated problems occur, it will be difficult to verify and justify the decisions an AI has made. An example made in the note, originally raised by the UK's House of Lords Select Committee, is that if AI is trained with data that doesn't represent a whole population, AI could wind up making discriminatory, unfair choices. Indeed, if AI is taught ineffectively, or if data is erroneous or outdated, then such a system could do more harm than good.

Another interesting point in the note was about how AI could cause isolation if it is used as a point of contact instead of a healthcare professional, especially if AI is brought into home healthcare and hospice situations. However, Nuffield Council on Bioethics also mentions the advantages of AI in-home treatment, especially in maintaining a patient's independence and quality of life.

Hugh Whittall, Director of the Nuffield Council, summarizes the main message perfectly: "The challenge [of AI] will be to ensure that innovation in AI is developed and used in ways that are transparent, that address societal needs, and that are consistent with public values." In short, AI can be a boon in the healthcare field, but it will be incomplete unless it possesses certain characteristics, such as human compassion too.

"Whether we are based on carbon or on silicon makes no fundamental difference; we should each be treated with appropriate respect."

- Arthur C. Clarke

PRESENT STATE & FUTURE OF AI IN MAJOR HEALTHCARE SPECIALTIES

CHAPTER NINE

PREVENTIVE HEALTHCARE

In the early 2000s, Google co-founder Larry Page[1] made an interesting prediction:

"Artificial intelligence would be the ultimate version of Google. The ultimate search engine that would understand everything on the Web. It would understand exactly what you wanted, and it would give you the right thing."

Twenty years later, the latest buzzwords in healthcare are Big Data and Artificial Intelligence (AI). Research shows that the field will see the growth of CAGR[2], which may reach 40% by 2024, giving rise to a 10-billion-dollar market focused on the different routes through which AI can impact healthcare delivery. These include broad-ranging fields, from medical imaging and radiology to lab medicine, diagnostics, genomics, personalized drug delivery, and even robotic AI assistants, through advanced Machine Learning, Deep Learning, and cognitive computing.

When Larry Page said that AI was the "ultimate search engine," he was referring to the fact that AI algorithms can process large amounts of data, analyzing them to give smart, actionable solutions. This has proved highly effective in the healthcare space. The 2020 pandemic has shown the global dearth of qualified and skilled healthcare personnel. The goal of using AI-based tools is to alleviate the cognitive burden of repetitive mundane tasks in order to free up healthcare workers so that they can focus on patient care, using their manual dexterity and skills. However, researchers soon discovered the untapped potential that AI offers, with solutions that can transform healthcare from a reactionary service to a preventive service.

All too often, patients are diagnosed with chronic conditions like endocrine issues or neoplasms simply because they missed symptoms or a diagnosis was delayed. This could be due to various reasons, but most research has delved into the ways in which patients can be diagnosed for health conditions at the earliest so that both curative and preventive measures can be taken to prevent mortality and morbidity, which may result from debilitative and costly late treatment measures. Studies have demonstrated that if patients have access to their own health data and if they are able to receive insights and feedback into their own health conditions, they are more willing to actively track their status and make lifestyle choices that are better for their health conditions. This concept ranges from routine monitoring of health parameters to active diagnosis and post-treatment evaluations.

The idea of remote patient monitoring seemed especially attractive in light of social distancing measures imposed by the 2020 pandemic. Patients were unable to visit treating physicians and depended on telehealth consultations, which, again, relied on health data collected by the patient himself through remote and user-friendly "wearable" devices. This large data set could reach treating physicians with the help of integrated smartphone applications, making it possible for real-time diagnosis and interventions. The large amount of data that was generated with remote monitoring devices were optimal for the application and training of AI-based algorithms. This could lead to machine-derived, predictive inferences, which in turn, would lead to personalized and preventive care for patients, catching disease symptoms earlier and more accurately.

If one plays devil's advocate, it is natural to ask: Can machines genuinely learn to think like doctors and surgeons? The multitude of research-based experimentation has answered that question with a resounding "yes." AI-based tools have already enhanced many healthcare branches by enabling doctors to make educated decisions, consultations, and interventions.

How AI is Revolutionizing Preventive Healthcare Now

Preventive healthcare has come into the limelight this past couple of years, especially as more people have called for an end to curative care. Stopping diseases and ailments before they have a chance to progress is critical to maintaining the health and well-being of any community. Thus, as healthcare is being reformed throughout the world, AI is offering modalities to get the job done. Thousands of startups working out AI for healthcare have popped up. These applications range from productivity in the office to enhancing the visuals of MRI scans and beyond. The best part is that both healthcare professionals and patients will have access to the data that AI will use, considering that the availability of knowledge is one of the most integral points of preventive care. Several healthcare IT applications are powered by AI, seeking to enhance patient care by reducing delays in treatment and highlighting risk factors within patients.

IBM Watson

Watson is famous for a number of interactions with humans, but its applications in healthcare are truly revolutionary. IBM created a special version of the *AI for oncologists*[3] to analyze and diagnose cancer states. It was found to be "concordant with the tumor board recommendations in 90 percent of breast cancer cases." With the multidisciplinary tumor board from India, Watson was concordant 96 percent for lung cancer, 81 percent for colon cancer, and 93 percent for rectal cancer. Now, Watson has become a reliable companion for oncologists throughout the world.

IBM Watson has also been used to power *Medtronic's IQ cast software*[4], which used the AI technology to train the application's *Sugar.IQ virtual* bot assistant to predict a patient's sugar level forecast, giving warnings for expected or sudden fluctuations in blood sugar levels and giving patients and physicians time to take interventions.

Healint

The main focus of the *Healint technology is* the *"Migraine Buddy" function*[5] that tracks migraines and keeps a diary. This data is analyzed using deep analytics and Machine Learning to give alerts on patient symptoms as well as medication results. The user can record the symptoms they get from their medication, which are sent to their treating physicians, who can then proactively adapt the treatment for such ailments.

What Can We Expect in the Future?

Every day, a discovery is made that will contribute to the healthcare of tomorrow. Aside from the benefits that are already obvious within the aforementioned examples, the advantages of incorporating AI into preventive healthcare are numerous. Here are just a few ways that AI is boosting the efficiency of the medical world for the present and future.

More Efficient Research Tools

Google and its parent company, Alphabet, are investing heavily in AI-based technology with a special focus on healthcare. Their subsidiary Verily is spearheading these attempts with data collecting research and analytics tools. Verily has focused its efforts on collaborating with medical research institutions around the world to find areas where they can apply AI-based solutions to capture biometric or health sensory data. Its wearable patient monitoring device, *the Study Watch*[6], is currently being used in clinical research programs as a prescription-only device to monitor patient conditions remotely for use in large population-based health trials as an easy way to accumulate data. They also introduced the *Verily Patch*[7], which is a novel sensor-based adhesive patch that can measure body temperature over long periods of time. It can be worn comfortably on the body continuously for up to 3 months. Another Alphabet subsidiary, Calico, is focusing on research into age-related diseases. It applies its algorithm to analyze large data sets and automate lab processes for faster diagnosis.

Better Data Management

AI can do something that humans can't—sift rapidly through data without getting distracted. In other words, AI will have access to billions of electronic medical records, scientific data, and other databases and will be able to find patterns and connections that humans may overlook.

*Waqaas Al-Siddiq, founder and CEO of **Biotricity**, states that AI's learning algorithms can "be deployed to traverse massive amounts of data and detect a few variables across hundreds of thousands of data points that are specific to certain conditions and diseases."*

Furthermore, fusing AI with blockchain technologies could enhance data management. An example would be **DeepMind Health**, another Google or Alphabet-owned enterprise that is leveraging AI for better health outcomes. Their algorithm mines data from medical records and expedites the treatment process. Most recently, through their **Alpha Fold** system, they have made computational-based predictions of the protein structures belonging to the COVID-19 virus, which will help in drug discovery research.[8]

Another system, called **Doc.ai**[9], uses blockchain to "collect masses of medical data globally" to generate individualized insights to patients for personalized medical aid.

Faster Online Consultations

The greatest asset AI brings to preventive healthcare is providing people with medical aid anywhere, anytime. As long as one has access to a cell phone connection or Wi-Fi, AI makes it possible to get consultations. An example of this is **Babylon**[10], an application that offers online consultations based on patients' individual medical records and medical databases. Users can input their data, report their illnesses, and receive feedback from the algorithm. The app also has functions like medication reminders and follow-ups that ask how you are feeling.

Similarly, **Engagely.ai**[11] provides personalized and accurate patient engagement by enabling physicians to diagnose with informed judgments. It also offers patients the right tools to make knowledge and evidence-based decisions about their health.

In the future, we can expect AI to grow more helpful with how it scans patients and gathers information. For example, a system called **AiCure**[12] is being developed by the National Institute of Health to use a smartphone's webcam to check up on patients, ensure that they are taking their prescriptions properly, and monitor a patient's overall condition, thereby helping doctors keep in touch with those who are having life-threatening conditions.

Conclusion

Artificial intelligence might seem like a futuristic concept, but it is here now, currently being used in wide-scale applications that most of us would be unaware of. With a number of algorithms being developed that learn how to think like a doctor, as well as with the automation of workflow, the creation of new medications, direct medical consultations, and better treatments, AI is fine-tuning healthcare daily. AI and medical professionals can now work together to create a more efficient system that stops ailments before they begin and treats patients quickly and more effectively than ever before. An exciting future with AI awaits.

References/Further Reading

Go to URL	Scan with a
MedMantra.com/a26	smartphone camera

CHAPTER TEN

NUTRITION

In the modern world, diet is important. People are becoming much concerned about their health and wish to maintain a nutritious diet that helps them sustain their wellbeing. But the question arises: what is 'healthy'?

On some days, the Paleo diet is proclaimed as the best thing for your body. On others, there is the Ketogenic diet that has become a trend rather quickly.

While some diets are said to be beneficial on a day – eventually, they may be declared detrimental. Not only does this variation exist between specific diets, but it also exists in essential everyday foods that we consume regularly. Foods like eggs and coffee may be considered healthy today, but you could be reading a headline tomorrow that tells you to avoid them at all costs.

At this stage, consumers are confused. People find themselves in a dilemma regarding which diet to follow or who to listen to. But here is the unfortunate truth: each body is unique. The idea that a specified diet would be healthy for every human is biologically impossible[1] – mainly since the way our food affects us differs on an individual level.

To break free of this struggle to determine the best diet for ourselves, we turn towards technology. More specifically, we look towards artificial intelligence.

Artificial Intelligence

Technology has become an integral part of our survival as human beings. We are beginning to rely more on technological advancements to aid our existence with each passing day. As a result, societies are also evolving.

The latest type of modern technology that has integrated itself into human lives is artificial intelligence. With the widespread launch of smartphone applications such as Siri or Cortana, there is increased access towards the world of artificial intelligence.[2]

But how does that impact or benefit us?

Well, with AI voice assistants around your home and your phones, there is so much that you can achieve. Most importantly, you could ask them a simple question: What should I eat?

AI and the Food Industry

Food is essential for human survival, and now, so is technology. The importance of AI in the food industry dates back to a few years ago when multinational companies such as IBM invested in using AI to create practical solutions for food-related problems.[3]

For instance, IBM is actively involved in research that includes the use of AI to pair various ingredients to develop new flavors and recipes for people. This research could prove to be a significant breakthrough for the food industry – since creating an entirely new flavor can be considered both scientific and artistic.[3] Since the process was too lengthy and too complicated for humans, IBM decided to leave all the work to artificial intelligence.[3]

AI in the food industry has proven to be quite efficient. It can make quick calculations and analyses based on the data collected and make corresponding changes immediately.

By using AI to develop new flavors by identifying patterns and considering alternatives, there are many new avenues now ready to be explored. Lucky for us, that includes an individualized diet-plan or the AI diet.

The AI Diet

Artificial intelligence can be used to create a perfect algorithm that tells you what to eat.[4] Since all of AI's suggestions are based on research and calculations, there is no doubt in believing that an AI diet could help people become healthier and significantly reduce their risk of getting a disease.

But why do we need an AI diet? Don't we already know the difference between healthy and unhealthy eating habits?

The truth is, we don't.

Dr. Eric Topol, a renowned cardiologist, participated in a 14-day experiment that involved tracking his dietary consumption, sleeping habits, and physical exercise. A sensor that tracked blood-glucose levels was provided, and a stool sample was also taken to assess his gut microbiome. After comparing his data with more than 1000 other participants' input, AI was able to create a personalized healthy/unhealthy grading scale for him.[5]

The results were anything but ordinary. The cheesecake was allocated an A grade in the sweets section, but whole-wheat fig bars were given a C. In fruits, strawberries were given an A+, while grapefruit was an unhealthy C. Apart from that, assorted nuts were given an A+ grade, but vegetable burgers had a C.[5]

Despite being a health practitioner, the results contradicted his existing beliefs regarding healthy eating. While his current diet was somewhat healthy, according to him, consisting of veggie burgers and whole-wheat fig bars, his nutritional intake wasn't actually healthy at all.[5]

As a result of this research, he realized that he had been eating unhealthy for the majority of his life. To avoid glucose spikes in the future, he was required to make significant changes to his diet – including integrating cheesecake and strawberries.

The main takeaway from this research was that humans are vastly unaware of what is healthy or unhealthy for their bodies. However, AI can help you determine a diet plan that is individualized and suited to your own biology – something that differs significantly from popular beliefs regarding healthy eating.

AI and Dietary Habits: Initial Developments

To successfully program AI to determine our individualized diet plans, we must first know why such variance exists in the first place. In simpler terms, why is something healthy for me but unhealthy for you?

The first significant development regarding this area of research was made a few years ago at the Weizmann Institute of Science. A journal article titled "Personalized Nutrition by Prediction of Glycemic Responses" was published, including the research that the spike in blood glucose levels as a response to consuming certain foods is only one aspect of our individualized responses towards nutrition.[6]

During this research, scientists made use of machine learning – a specialized branch of artificial intelligence that focuses on patterns. The goal was to determine the critical factor that drove the blood-glucose response towards food for each individual.

After analyzing billions of possible factors, the research was concluded with about a hundred factors that were actively involved in this glycemic response in humans. Instead of the key factor being food itself, it was actually concluded to be the gut bacteria – or microbiome.

As a result of this research, two conclusions were made. One that our microbiome is mainly responsible for our spike in blood glucose levels, and two, that this groundbreaking discovery was only made using AI.[6]

For continued development, more research is underway to determine the different biological responses our bodies have towards the same kinds and amounts of food.[7,8] The fascinating part, however, that all of these researches now include AI to analyze the large amount of data being collected and to reach evidence-based results.

The Importance of Biotechnology

In order to successfully generate all of these personalized AI diets we keep referring to, there needs to be a method of handling big data. This process requires many different technologies to be combined into one major development – something that is beyond the expertise of nutritionists or the food industry.

This brings us to the need for development in biotechnology – or the application of modern technology in the creation of individualized diets. AI diets require chunks of data on both life and diet habits, which comes together under the branch of biotechnology[9] due to its close relationship with life sciences.

In simpler terms, the future of an AI diet could stand on the foundations of modern biotechnology. Since an effective AI mechanism to generate customized diet plans requires the filtering of fake data as well as the simultaneous processing of different information, biotechnology is the only branch of science that would be able to aid the process seamlessly.

The Problem with Fake Data

On the topic of how biotechnology aids the process of having an AI diet, it is also vital to understand what nutritional science lacks at the moment. While many people believe that our diet and health are interconnected, the connection is overly complicated.

Without using modern biotechnology or AI, it is nearly impossible to conduct randomized trials at large scales. Observing the effects of a specific diet may span for many years before any conclusion can be drawn – and such close adherence to a diet and tracking of behavior is rarely ever controlled.

As a result of these imperfect researches, there is a great deal of fake data available regarding dietary habits and nutrition.[10] For instance, if you look at the oxalate quantities in different foods, the values you find will vary significantly from one source to another.[11] The difference could be so vast that while one article would suggest a particular food to be great for your health, another would advise you to remove it from your diet altogether.

Our Diets Are Flawed: The Evidence

Before resorting to AI for customized diets, it is important to consider the various researches that have already concluded that our diets are extremely flawed. The main reason for the flaw, however, is the amount of fake data available to us regarding 'healthy' and 'unhealthy' eating habits.

Depending on which source we choose to follow, we could have a completely different belief system regarding the contents of certain foods. Consequently, we could be eating less or more of a certain food without having any concrete evidence regarding its effect on our body.

A 2017 study conducted in the US investigated the consumption of 10 specific foods in more than half a million people who died from heart disease.[12] In the research, diets that consisted of salty foods and processed meats were considered to have adverse outcomes. A similar strategy was used for other kinds of foods as well.

With "convincing" evidence, the study concluded that 45% of the deaths were due to the ten dietary factors being researched.[12] In simpler words, it was concluded that half of all deaths from heart disease are caused by a poor or unbalanced diet.

Similar studies related to diet and fatality have made conclusions such as that plant-based diets can lessen the chance of developing type 2 diabetes[13] and that regular consumption of whole-grain foods can result in lower cases of heart disease or cancer.[14]

However, there is a major flaw in all of these studies: the dependency on self-reporting. Participants may not have accurately reported their dietary and other habits, resulting in an influx of false information. Additionally, these researches also do not have any controls and fail to eliminate confounding factors such as socioeconomic environments or literacy rates.

Consequently, such researches that are low in reliability still make their way to the public in the form of media headlines or journal articles – thus impacting the kinds of diet, we consume. Depending upon the day, every type of food ends up labeled both helpful and harmful.

The Problem with a Fixed Diet

As a result of fake news that circulates based on flawed research, many problems arise with our typical fixed diet. The idea of collectively following a specific nutritional guideline is both biologically and physiologically flawed, especially since it fails to consider the individuality of each human body.

In all individuals, there are varying metabolisms, microbiome, and external environments that contribute towards their physiological reaction towards food.[15] Despite consuming the same amount of the same food at the same time, it is possible and highly likely for two people to have varying biological reactions.

This can be attributed to many factors, including how our unique DNA can react to foods in varying manners.

Solving the Problem with Modern Biotechnology

Since our bodies react to foods in different ways, it can be useful to understand what aspects of our DNA differ and how the use of biotechnology with AI can help us find a solution to the problem.

1. Whole Genome Sequence Analysis

With modern biotechnology, science can analyze a person's entire genome and further understand how specific genes are related to certain diseases.[16] By analyzing the genetic compound of a person, it is possible to create a customized nutrition plan that is in accordance with their bodily functions and helps them avoid the instance of illness.

2. Nutrigenetics

Contrary to popular belief that the only way food impacts our bodies is through the nutrients it contains, modern biotechnology has now proven that food has a significant influence on DNA expressions that impact an individual's health.[17] With these technologies, it is possible to understand the varying health effects of consuming certain foods with relevance to genetic expressions – thus allowing AI to gather data and create customized dietary plans.

3. Proteomics

The tRNA signal transduction system in our body is greatly affected by the food we eat[18], which could result in certain proteomes being synthesized. Since these proteomes are essential for bodily functions such as growth and balance, the data collected through DNA expression can be used to determine healthier food choices.

4. Nutrigenomics

The genetic structure of each individual is different. While food impacts our genetic expression, our varying genetic structures also lead to different metabolomic reactions within the body. This nutrigenomic data is, therefore, necessary during the creation of smart, AI diets.[19]

5. Metabolomics

While not causally related to food consumption, metabolomic data is still essential for the creation of AI diets since it allows for a deeper understanding of how overall lifestyle (sleep, exercise) impacts the health of an individual.[19]

6. Microbiome

Multiple studies have concluded that the food we consume affects not only our gene expression but also the gut bacteria that live inside our bodies.[20] While food does not change the DNA of gut bacteria, it does cause significant changes in the microbiome. This microbiome is related to both health and immunity – the two things that are the critical determinants for developing a good diet.

The Amalgamation of AI and What We Eat

In the present world, a popular food company was able to integrate AI with the food that is consumed by their customers. They introduced what is known as LIFEdata solutions[21] that are meant to engage with customers throughout the day to develop healthy eating habits that are customized for the specific user.

The platform works by understanding the user's lifestyle habits, external environment, motivational factors, and behavioral changes that go hand-in-hand with dietary habits. While it is not perfect, the platform currently has a mobile app that contains an entire database of nutritional data, varying recipes, and an integrated AI to provide smart suggestions.

The recommendations made to each user are based upon several self-report data inputs, including common surveys and detailed medical histories. By combining all of this data with eating habits and physiological reactions, personalized recommendations are made regarding dietary habits for each individual user.

Important features of this app include a simple method of selection between the correct food consumption to teach smart eating habits to children and entire families – based on their current medical and food consumption data. By following the smart suggestions provided by the AI, people can easily prevent chronic illnesses and choose to consume food that is especially healthy for their bodies.

Apart from that, the app also includes a voice assistant that can help people find recipes according to what they have available in their kitchens, as well as a step-by-step guide for recipe preparation.

The Mechanism of AI-Guided Diet Plans

Similar to the practical example of an AI-based solution quoted above, the mechanism of an AI-guided diet plan would also rely on machine learning and data analytics. With a deep understanding of the users' metabolic and digestive systems, the AI-based diet plan would be able to provide suggestions for ideal meals that would help your body rejuvenate.

This personalized diet plan is likely to contain the ability to save millions of lives per year. With diets that are specific to our bodily functions, preventing chronic illnesses such as diabetes, cancer, or heart disease would become much simpler.

Additionally, since many people resort to strict diets to lose weight, an AI-based solution will be much more effective in that aspect as well. By making use of big data and biotechnology, the AI-based diet plan would have a 72% probability of helping you lose weight.[22]

However, there is a critical downside to the use of AI-based diet plans that must be considered. Thousands of nutritionists across the globe may find themselves jobless if an AI-based diet plan system proves itself to be more efficient than these health practitioners. The likelihood of efficiency is extremely high in AI-based diet plans, especially since these machine learning systems will be able to process millions of bits of data within seconds[22] – something that the human mind cannot independently achieve.

Nevertheless, there is still an opportunity for existing nutritionists to expand their skillset and familiarize themselves with the applications of AI in the nutritional world. This would allow them to help people understand how the AI-based diet plans work and enabling users to make the most efficient use of such applications.

AI and Nutrition: The Future

While there are some developments in the field of AI for the food industry, they are definitely far from perfect. There are many more research areas that are yet to be covered before any significant developments can be made for customized diets using modern biotechnology as well as the different branches of AI.

However, there is no denying the usefulness of integrating AI with nutrition. In fact, an individualized and tailored diet will be able to promote a healthy lifestyle and allow our virtual assistants to take on a more significant role in our lives.

While a majority of AI-related dietary plans are still in their initial development stages, it is safe to say that technological advancement is fast enough for us to be soon testing personalized diet plans for ourselves.

We cannot know for sure what the future will bring for the food industry, especially with biotechnology and AI on the line now. However, we are certainly on the path towards creating increased access to legitimate information regarding dietary habits and implementing significant lifestyle changes. Hopefully, with AI-based diets, we would all be able to live healthier, happier, and longer lives.

References/Further Reading

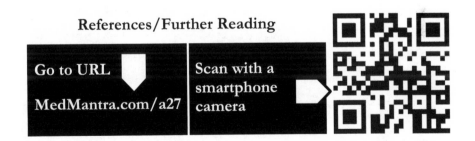

Go to URL
MedMantra.com/a27

Scan with a smartphone camera

CHAPTER ELEVEN
RADIOLOGY

One of the important specialties of healthcare, radiology, is no stranger to involvement in medical advancements and AI integration. For many years now, computers have been an essential part of radiology. Therefore, it is no surprise that AI is now analyzing x-rays, CT scans, MRIs, and the like for abnormal readings, just like a radiologist would.

Yet, this also raises several questions about the future of radiology and just how important AI is to the progression of healthcare. In what ways can AI boost diagnostic efficacy in the radiology field? Will AI automate the tasks of radiologists? Will it be accurate and precise? One thing is certain: AI epitomizes potential for vastly improving medical examinations and diagnoses.

The Present State of Machine Learning in Clinical Imaging

Even with many start-ups or established research centers developing comprehensive AI-based tools for radio-imaging, it may be beneficial to understand how many of these applications are finally applied in the field and whether they really deliver the solutions they promised, outside of a trial set up.

A recent meta-analysis conducted by Rezazade M. and colleagues for the European Radiology Journal in 2020 evaluated all AI applications presented at the RSNA (Radiological Society of North America), ECR (European Congress of Radiology), and SIIM (Society for Imaging Informatics in Medicine) from 2017 to 2019, as well as trial studies and market research reports. They analyzed data from various sources to determine functionalities, focal modalities, targeted steps in the workflows, anatomical regions, and developmental and regulatory approval phases.

While North America and Europe took up most of the market share, at 41% and 22%, respectively, Asian companies also showed predominance, at 19%. Most of the applications are approved by the FDA or CE, while some countries, like Canada and Korea, have their own regulations for medical device approval. Fifty-four percent are built to retrofit with existing

PACS/RIS systems, while 25% are stand-alone. Seventy-four percent of the AI-based software analyzed was applied to CT, MRI, and X-ray images, while only 17% were meant to be applied in USG or mammography images. Breast screening data and diseases like the Big 3—lung cancer, COPD, and cardiovascular diseases—as well as brain imaging, are usually the focus of large-scale studies, and there has been tremendous growth in applications for the diagnosis of these conditions.

Eighty-seven percent of the AI-based algorithms are built to target reasoning and perception during the radiology workflow, that is, on improving the efficiency and speed of reporting images or scans.

Therefore, there is room to develop systems that help with areas like administration, the acquisition of machines, the processing of good-quality images, and transcription and reporting. Algorithms can be used to develop clinical decision-making support tools to determine which radiological investigations or radiation contrast dosages may be applied to individuals with common presenting features of conditions. Others may be used to monitor the downtime of machines, as well as maintenance or repair time, and to schedule tasks to balance the workload of the radiologists. Automated and AI-enhanced image processing enables clear, bright, and good-resolution images to be taken without skilled labor and without repetition, reducing the radiation exposure for patients and saving time for medical staff, with overall improved efficiency in operations. These innovations would truly make the applications of AI and machine learning systems in the field of radiology more comprehensive.[1]

Current Applications of AI-Based Radiology Systems

In 2015, a start-up based in San Francisco, *Enlitic*, flew software engineers to 80 clinical imaging centers throughout Central Asia, South East Asia, and Australia. These software engineers brought with them deep learning (AI) algorithm that had been designed to integrate with PACS, otherwise known as picture archiving and communication systems. Enlitic aims to use the algorithm to identify early stages of disease during clinical imaging sessions, including nuclear medicine, ultrasound, X-ray, computed tomography (CT), and magnetic resonance imaging (MRI). In 2016, Enlitic conducted a study that proved its AI software can improve the detection accuracy of radiologists in search of extremity fractures. According to its findings, the use of the Enlitic machine learning software alone aided in a 20% improvement in efficiency.[2]

Enlitic isn't the only up-and-coming software company with a hand in healthcare. Another San Francisco-based company, named *Arterys*, is making waves with its machine learning software. In November 2016, the FDA granted 501(k) clearance for Arterys 4D Flow software. 4D Flow is presently being used in cardiac MRI studies to improve the overall visualization and quantification of blood flow.[3]

In January 2017, another program, *Cardio DL*, was given the same clearance level. Similar to 4D Flow, Cardio DL is a cloud-based image processing technology that uses machine learning for the identification and segmentation of cardiac ventricles.[4]

To construct 4D Flow, Arterys formed a partnership with *Vios Works by GE Healthcare*. Arterys blended its cloud processing with the GE software for MRI machines. Though the product has not yet been released, already more than 40 hospitals are using the 4D Flow system for their research and have successfully used it in more than 10,000 cases.[5]

A Silicon Valley company called *RADLogics* is noted for creating *Alpha Point* software, a program that utilizes machine learning in preliminary findings, such as how a doctor would use medical records information and analyze the images from a radiology report. Already, the software has been given FDA clearance for chest CT scans and has been validated for chest X-rays. RADLogics is currently pursuing clearance for MRI scans as well.

During the 2020 Covid-19 pandemic, RADLogics deployed its AI-powered imaging software to analyze CT scans and X-rays from hospitals and clinics in the United States, Russia, Europe, China, and India, which greatly helped with patient triaging and rapid management. The application allowed for quantitative analysis of images, which could integrate seamlessly with existing software, making it scalable and offering global reach. Its accuracy has been validated in multiple clinical studies and, due to the rich influx of patient-related data, the machine learning algorithm has continued to improve and evolve.[6]

The co-founder of RADLogics, Moshe Becker, has stated that the software is meant to remove time-consuming measurements and other grunt work from the radiologist's workload. In fact, the software is more or less a virtual assistant. "Radiologists are valuable as diagnosticians. But, just as humans aren't that great in pixel counting or being a visual search engine, we're helping them go through the work more accurately, more consistently, and saving time." In fact, helping radiologists has become the company's primary goal.[7]

Meanwhile, other companies that aren't inherently medical have also begun dabbling in the healthcare setting. For example, *IBM has been working with its Watson system* to create *Watson Health*, which helps physicians with their diagnoses. From America to China to Europe to India and beyond, groups are endeavoring to revolutionize medical imaging with artificial intelligence.[8]

CAR AI Working Group

One of the latest and most extensive research groups is the *Canadian Association of Radiologists (CAR)* and the *AI Working Group*, founded in May 2017. Members of the working group include those in both pediatric and adult radiology as well as specialties in informatics, biophysics, and other research areas. The idea was to "discuss and deliberate on practice, policy, and patient care issues related to the introduction and implementation of AI in imaging." The primary goal was that radiologists could work together with AI developers to influence the way that such technology impacts their roles in the healthcare field. Other objectives include:

- Considering the potential impact of AI on radiology in Canada.

- Developing CAR policy regarding the usage and deployment of AI systems.

- Promoting and facilitating research in areas such as improving computer-aided design (CAD) systems, radiomics, computer-assisted reporting, natural language processing, and more.

- Offering guidance and support to help members incorporate AI systems into their practices in a way that will benefit patients and employees, such as optimizing workflow.

- Studying how AI learns through extensive research in elements like deep/machine learning and AI neural pathways, which are developed by relaying slightly different bits of information to the algorithms, creating a machine version of neuroplasticity.

- Looking into the social and ethical issues that the medical field may have to confront with the growing usage of deep/machine learning in healthcare.

While researching AI in multiple pathways, as well as how the machine learning software can evolve under certain conditions, the AI Working Group posed a powerful question: What is the impact of AI on radiology? Presently, AI is heavily impacting PACS, especially for tasks that are "prone to human error," such as detecting lung nodules (lung cancer) on X-rays or bone metastases on computed tomography (CT) scans. The working group concluded that while AI can improve the performance of clinicians, it cannot replace medical professionals. Another observation was that the pairing between clinician or physician and AI was better than either entity working alone.[9]

With this line of thinking, perhaps other countries should be establishing working groups for official radiology associations and allowing them to have a say in how AI is being integrated into the field. When miraculous medical advances are being made that benefit both physician and patient, and when radiologists are coming to realize that AI is not jeopardizing their position, better care can be delivered to patients worldwide.

How AI Will Change Radiology

One of the biggest challenges in the healthcare field presently is the amount of data being heaped on top of an already overwhelming workload for physicians and clinicians, including radiologists. Although electronic medical records (EMRs) have saved hospitals and doctors' offices from being flooded with papers and files, there are still exams, procedure reports, lab readings, EKG scans, pathology reports, and so much more. Through all of this raw data, medical professionals are expected to find the answer to a patient's discomfort.

That is where AI will change the entire healthcare industry, radiology included. Though AI cannot replace a human in many facets of healthcare, it can boost innate human comprehension to accelerate the discovery of the root cause of a patient's illness or pain. For example, a patient might be having chest pain. AI can look at computed tomography (CT) scan and single out the most relevant cause—or provide a narrowed-down number of possibilities. Thus, AI systems will improve medical imaging by doing the following:

- Scouring relevant data from prior medical exams with a focus on cardiac history.

- Looking into pharmacy information for drugs related to heart failure, coronary disease, COPD, and anticoagulants.

- Looking at previous chest CT scans to aid in analysis, including previous patient records, procedures, lab results, and pathology reports from similar cases.

In the end, the AI system might correctly weigh various causes that the doctors had been considering and put them on the right path. Without the aid of the AI system going through all this data within seconds, the patient's condition and health would worsen during the wait. In short, where humans are slow in scanning data and finding the answer, a computer can swiftly find the patterns and most probable causes.

A study was published in the *Public Library of Science* that reported on the development of a "collective intelligence" of radiologists that reduced the number of false positives and false negatives when reading mammograms. The Swarm AI was able to overcome "one of the fundamental limitations to decision accuracy that individual radiologists face," the researchers concluded. In other words, this "swarm intelligence" allowed groups of experts to come together and improve their decision-making skills. Everyone in the medical field knows that completing something a few seconds sooner can be lifesaving.[10]

Of course, AI will change the effectiveness of medical diagnosis in other ways, too. As seen with Arterys and Enlitic technologies, AI has already become an asset in radiology because it can accurately classify normal and abnormal MRI scans and x-rays with the same accuracy as a human. It doesn't matter if the clinical imaging is focused on intervertebral discs, torn ligaments, or cancer nodules—AI is capable of detecting these issues and reporting them to the radiologist. Not only does this improve the quality of the report, but it also improves the overall quality of care.

Why Radiologists Need AI

Going back to Enlitic for a moment—during the research, the engineers at Enlitic found that radiologists were hesitant to adopt the AI system. For example, during a lung cancer screening product trial, the radiologists would often overlook the analysis of the AI and instead use textbooks in search of rare cases. The Enlitic engineers noted how much time searching textbooks for information could take. When the AI system was used, however, the machine learning software would look for a history of lung nodules that were characteristically similar to what had been found on the image and make an appropriate detection that much faster.

There are more advantages to merging AI with medical imaging, though. Some of those benefits have been covered. Others are less apparent.

Let's take a moment to consider the experiences of **Mark Michalski, MD**, executive director of the *Brigham & Women's Hospital Center (BWH) for Clinical Data Science and the Massachusetts General Hospital (MGH)*. Michalski believes that AI can become the companion that radiologists have always needed—and sooner rather than later.[11]

In 2016, MGH paired up with **Nvidia,** an internationally renowned technology company, to employ a server made especially for AI applications called **DGX-1**. The MGH data scientists and Nvidia engineers were able to implement deep learning algorithms that took in 10 billion images from MGH records for training. Though much of the AI system is still in its infancy, the main algorithm that is being readily utilized is one to help radiologists assess bone age. How was it done? After exposing the deep learning algorithm to a plethora of (already interpreted) images related to bone age, it was able to learn how to conduct a satisfactory assessment. Now, radiologists enthusiastically use the AI system to aid them in their readings.[12]

Beyond having the benefit of an assistant that can carry out accurate assessments and enhance images, there is also the buzzword "automation" to think about. Many might recoil at the sight and sound of the word, but, in reality, automation goes hand in hand with AI. *Joerg Aumuller* from the *Artificial Intelligence and Decision Support Solutions department* at **Siemens Healthineers** stated, "The average radiologist is forced to interpret images quickly, potentially reducing diagnostic accuracy. When radiologists are rushed, their error rate rises... AI combines human and machine to be more powerful than the human alone".[13]

While the above statement is a nod toward the aspirations of swarm AI and software like RADLogics, one cannot overlook the main advantage: smoother workflow. For instance, AI could review chest X-rays and abnormalities in organs, and highlight these abnormal regions ahead of time, which would give the radiologist more time to study the images in full. An excellent example of this is the algorithm developed by **Predible Health (Bengaluru, India)** that can detect liver tumors. Without the AI, the time associated with segmenting out liver vessels, parenchyma, and tumors would be 45-60 minutes. Use of the AI dropped that time down to 5-10 minutes, leading to a faster diagnosis. The company worked with hospitals in India to access a rich mine of patient data in order to train the AI algorithm to develop two real-time applications. The first one is Predible Liver, which helps with the accurate planning that surgeons carry out before liver transplants or neoplasm resections. The second one, Predible Lung, accelerated lung nodule interpretation in CT scan images. Research is ongoing to introduce a platform for rapid stroke detection.[14]

AI vs. Radiologists

Naturally, these recent advancements in AI throughout several industries have raised the question of whether or not AI will one day completely automate the healthcare industry. In other words, will radiology become a job of a forgotten age? While it might seem that AI could overwhelm the healthcare field, it will not erase radiologists. Rather, it will enhance the efficacy of X-ray and MRI images, allowing radiologists to make more precise readings and analyses. However, before getting into why radiologists should be welcoming AI advancements rather than fearing them, we will review a few reasons why AI will change radiology for the better:

1. Humans Will Always Be Responsible

Despite automation's evolution throughout the years, it is mankind's desire for safety and communication. In other words, when legal responsibility is attached to the care of a patient, there is no fathomable circumstance in which the AI unit itself will be held accountable for a mistake. Someone must be there to take responsibility and offer recompense in some way. This means that it will always fall upon a human to check the analysis an AI system has made and finalize the decision. Although AI will aid the radiologist in developing clearer, more precise imaging, the AI system itself will be incapable of answering medical diagnostic questions 100% of the time.

2. Radiologists Look at More Than Images

Because radiology is more than looking at a single picture, there are dozens of tasks that an AI system cannot do. Many of these duties are designed for a human only. For example, a radiologist has face-to-face time with patients (such as discussing medical history details and providing directions during the examination period), must calibrate the machine and properly set the measurements, and must know how to choose the correct image type every time. Radiologists must also be able to identify certain types of readings (such as nodule detection or a hemorrhage), consult other physicians about diagnosis and treatment options, provide patient care (such as local ablative therapy), perform interventional radiology procedures, and tailor settings to a patient's condition. These are all things that only a flesh-and-blood person can do because they require emotional intelligence—which AI doesn't have—and hands-on action.

3. Machine Learning Takes Time

As mentioned previously in the section explaining the objective of the CAR AI Working Group, AI is not automatically all-knowing when it comes to the task it has been given. There are deep learning algorithms that form the brain, and it must learn through a flow of data. Someone will have to be there to figuratively hold the AI's hand and show it the way. Because no database of X-ray images is available to dump into the AI's brain, every new system will be starting from zero. The often-overlooked benefit of this, however, is that more radiologists will have to be hired to deal with the images and data being fed into the machine, especially when demand for AI-enhanced X-rays and MRIs increases exponentially in the next few years.AI might be able to schedule appointments and interpret images, but that won't cover even half of what a radiologist does daily.

Artificial Intelligence in Interventional Radiology

What Is Interventional Radiology?

Interventional radiology (IR) is a subspecialty of radiology responsible for performing many minimally invasive procedures.[15] These procedures are performed under medical imaging guidance, including x-ray fluoroscopy, ultrasound, magnetic resonance imaging, and computed tomography.

The primary goal of IR is to treat patients using the least invasive procedures available in the healthcare world. This minimizes the risk to patients and enhances the outcomes. IR procedures result in less pain, less risk, and less recovery time compared to standard surgical procedures.[15]

By integrating machine learning (ML) into diagnosis and treatment, AI can change the game for IR. It will empower healthcare professionals to efficiently offer the highest-quality care. Through AI, Big Data can be quickly analyzed to uncover new insights that aid radiologists.

Applications of AI in IR

1. Forecasting Outcomes

The biggest challenge IR faces is that professionals can't forecast the outcomes of treatment before performing it. They must devise an accurate method with a high success rate to reduce unnecessary interventions and procedures. This also reduces healthcare costs and risks to the patient.

Treatment efficacy must be measured before the patient agrees to the treatment. Such a challenge can be overcome with the help of AI, mainly deep learning (DL). The baseline diagnostic images of a patient's clinical data, and the outcomes of the planned intervention, can be used to teach the AI to work on a model that can learn the relationship between these variables and the procedure results.[16]

The results of the model would enable the prediction of the procedure outcome in new patients. Keep in mind that the characteristics of the intervention must be specified to obtain accurate results. DL-based AI can help interventional radiologists during the decision-making process.

2. Improving the Diagnosis

Another important application of AI in IR is to improve clinical imaging diagnoses. This involves DL-based classification of images, which helps radiologists. CNNs, also known as convolutional neural networks, are used to classify the hepatic masses on MR imaging, CT, and even ultrasound scans.[17,18]

Besides that, the higher the use of CNNs in the field, the more that healthcare specialists will learn about them and utilize them to enhance the patient care quality in IR. Keep in mind that CNNs function primarily as a black box. That is why an approach incorporating interpretability of the outcomes will help with clinical translation by allowing healthcare professionals to understand why decisions were made and predict why a decision may fail.

Creating such a model is tantamount in the field of IR. That is because it will enhance workflow and help IR professionals identify novel imaging biomarkers for an accurate and effective diagnosis. Improved diagnoses can significantly transform IR for patients and healthcare professionals.

3. Enhancing IR Procedures

There is always room for improvement, especially in the field of healthcare. Even in IR, radiologists must overcome challenges like high costs, slow decision-making, and more. These procedures increase patients' wait time and treatment costs.

Once AI is introduced in IR on a large scale, these procedures will improve significantly. The primary aim of AI in the healthcare industry is to reduce costs. The aim can also be achieved in IR, such as by automating many imaging and decision-making processes to significantly cut down costs.

Besides that, AI can enhance different aspects of IR. For example, remote catheter navigation assistance systems have been developed to improve the experience of interventional radiologists. The CorPath GRX Vascular Robotic System by Corindus (a Siemens Healthineers company) provides precise (sub-millimeter precision) device positioning from a distance during interventional procedures.[19-21]

It offers robotic-assisted control of guide catheters, guidewires, and rapid exchange catheters and provides radiation protection to the IR physician, as well as potentially reduces radiation exposure to staff and patients. In the same way, many new technologies can be developed to enhance various IR procedures.

ML models can run and offer results in milliseconds. These can allow for computations that improve the timing of decision-making processes in the field of IR. In the long run, both the patients and the radiologists will benefit from improved turn-around time and procedures in the field of IR.

4. Enhancing Patient Selection

Finally, AI in IR is also capable of enhancing patient selection. That is because ML can help professionals predict therapeutic outcomes.[22] This means more patients going through procedures in IR will receive the quality care they need.

The best part about using an ML model is that fewer patients will be exposed to IR treatments that will not benefit them in any way.[16] Of course, that is just one way AI can improve IR when it comes to patient selection. The model can be expanded to many other cohorts to strengthen the entire process from diagnosis to treatment.

For example, before any therapy starts, AI mechanisms can identify nonresponders. When this happens, patients will be saved from unnecessary treatment and therapies. However, for the outcomes to be accurate, the AI must be fed with appropriate data.

Once the data is appropriate, the AI will make more accurate predictions and offer therapeutic recommendations that patients require. The data must also be validated and updated from time to time. Retraining the model is essential to get the most use out of it, as this affects the patients' experience when it comes to treatment.

Final Words – AI in IR

AI has many other potential applications in IR. Often, diagnostic radiologists are not available; this is an area that can drastically improve in the coming years. Besides that, AI has the power to provide higher quality care and a more accurate diagnosis.

Of course, AI techniques are at the stage where they are still evolving. The ethical problems involved in designing AI must be discussed and agreed upon by everyone involved in the process. In addition, more research is needed to create some of the best AI algorithms that the medical industry has ever seen.

Once all the proper steps have been followed, AI can drastically improve patient care and radiologist performance outcomes. The field of IR can significantly change once AI is in motion.

Conclusion

All in all, it is safe to say that the future of medicine and research lies in the virtual hands of deep/machine learning, also known as artificial intelligence. The revolution is happening now, all around us. Algorithms are interwoven into our daily lives, from Facebook's automatic face-tagging feature to the Amazon Alexa perched on the bookshelf. However, the biggest problem that AI faces is the hesitation of implementation that many medical professionals, including radiologists, have. Because many see AI as automation—and, thus, an adversary in the workforce—getting radiologists to adopt the technology that can help them is the current challenge.

What should be stressed is not the automation or how advanced the technology has already become, but how AI is more of an assistant that spots irregularities and reduces human error while simultaneously combining individual intelligence to accelerate diagnosis. AI will support radiologists in becoming a more evolved form of a medical professional than before, as they will have the time to completely examine the details of an image, communicate the results of the combined AI and radiologist findings, and play a more active role in the diagnosis of illness and disorders, as well as in the treatment of patients.

Perhaps, in the future, radiology and other medical fields will need to be renamed, but the human factor of healthcare will never change. The future of radiology lies within artificial intelligence, so let's allow AI to flourish and bring about a better future for everyone.

References/Further Reading

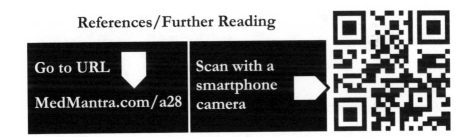

Go to URL	Scan with a smartphone camera
MedMantra.com/a28	

CHAPTER TWELVE

PATHOLOGY

To take medical diagnosis and research to the next level, the latest advancements in technology, such as artificial intelligence (AI) and machine learning (ML), have to be considered.

The focus of the AI industry has unsurprisingly been on the applications of clinical diagnostics in fields like pathology. The idea is simple - to handover repetitive and time-consuming tasks to a machine so that the human experts can focus on more challenging and complex cases.

Data shows that low-income and middle-income countries (LMICs), which have a disproportionately large share of the global burden of diseases, have an inversely low number of trained professionals who can contribute to laboratory medicine services.[1]

Pathologists are a relatively small population of medical professionals in the healthcare industry. They could largely benefit from the support that AI technology could provide in order to tackle the growing threat of stronger, more resilient diseases, pathogens, and non-infectious disorders. While other healthcare sectors have adopted AI to take on tasks like regulating workflow or scanning data, its implementation in pathology has been fairly recent. However, the benefits that this budding partnership has already provided are undeniable and have brought about rapid improvements in the field.

The Growth of Digital Pathology

Climate change, industrialization, and other factors have long influenced the diseases and pathogens that affect humankind. Due to rising cancer rates as well as incidences of non-communicable diseases leading to chronic health conditions, there is an urgency to adopt digital pathology in clinical fields, with the hope to improve existing diagnostic measures and reduce costs associated with conventional methods.

In 2019, the digital pathology market was determined to be USD 767.6 million worldwide. It is predicted to grow at an 11.8% compound annual growth rate (CAGR) from 2020 to 2027 due to efforts made to improve the efficiency of workflows leading to rapid diagnostic tools. The Asia Pacific region will show a faster rate of expansion, expected to be at 12.9%, because of the rising popularity of digital imaging in growing economies.[2]

Whole slide imaging (WSI) captures images of tissue microscopy and uploads them into databases with specialized scanners. These databases are studied and analyzed to come to a diagnosis. WSI allows pathologists to visualize the data on a computer screen or a virtual microscope that allows for improvements in education, training, diagnostics, consultations, meetings, archiving, and more. According to the traditional surgical pathology lab workflow, after manual sectioning, several slides from the tissue specimen are sliced, and additional special stains or immunohistochemistry tests are applied. With WSI, pathologists make a series of whole slide images to use along with textbooks, medical records, and other previously collected molecular or lab data. However, due to the sheer data size of slides (2-3GB per image), they must be processed using an updated digital workflow. The data sets formed are enormous, and here lies the natural progression towards AI to help with analysis.

The adoption of AI in digital pathology requires the slides to be imported into a software program, which uses machine learning to spot subtle patterns and provide detailed information to the pathologist. Not only can specimens be analyzed by AI from different angles, but the workflow is also streamlined, and thus the efficiency and efficacy in reporting and diagnosis are increased.

Current advancements include whole slide imaging and robotic light microscopy, backed by ambient computing through fiber-optic communications, which work together to improve the applications of digitalization in pathology. Predictive and hybrid models used along with micro-arrays lead to efficient computer-aided diagnosis, along with estimations of disease progression and risk assessments, resulting in improved research and treatment initiatives.

Why does Pathology Need AI and ML?

Presently, cancer affects 1 in every three persons globally, which means that by 2030, more than half of the entire planet's population will have some form of cancer. However, pathologists cannot keep up with the demand for body tissue samples that require study. China, for instance, has about 20,000 pathologists in the entire country, but given the size of the total population, over 100,000 pathologists would be required to handle the workload.

More importantly, pathologists are constrained to what the human eye can detect in tissue samples put underneath the lens of a microscope to recognize patterns and correlate them with clinical findings. Even with digital whole slide imaging and other ways to collect visual data, there is a limit to the kind of information pathologists can obtain, on their own, in a time-bound manner. On the other hand, AI will be able to look at the details from a multitude of different perspectives, accessing new information from a wide range of disparate healthcare and research databases – inside and outside individual facilities. As such, there will be analysis made on larger data sets, revealing previously unobtained useful conclusions that can help solve cases faster, enabling the pathologist to move on to another case, thereby improving turnaround time.

This amalgamation of advanced imaging, automation, and powerful analytics like natural language processing (NLP), machine learning, and artificial intelligence (AI) in the field is bringing together the tools needed for accelerated diagnosis and earlier treatment options for patients.

In 2018, the UK established *The Path LAKE Consortium* as one of its 5 AI centers of excellence funded by UK Research and Innovation (UKRI). It brought together university and NHS partners committed to the creation of completely digital cellular pathology laboratories, along with an ethically approved data lake of anonymous scanned slide images, used to train and develop AI algorithms.[3]

Another large-scale digital slide library is *The Cancer Genome Atlas,* which allows researchers to access a large database of annotated pathology images linked with clinical and genomic history, which acts as training material for AI-based software in pathology diagnosis.[4]

The Future of Artificial Intelligence in Pathology

Though pathology departments have already integrated faster and more powerful technologies into their laboratories, the most exciting time for artificial intelligence and pathology is on the horizon. Many of the advancements go beyond the usefulness of WSI by incorporating the latest algorithms from deep learning to enhance the diagnostic capabilities of AI systems. These Deep learning systems create the possibility of machine-aided pathology or Computer-Aided Diagnosis (CAD).

This means that AI will be able to aid the pathologist in the following sections of work:

1. Formulating a hypothesis

Currently, pathologists arrive at a hypothesis by going through a systematic process based on what they know. They ask themselves what is relevant, and depending on their experience; they may overlook other possibilities. With AI support, thousands of pieces of data (from electronic patient records, ECGs, EEGs, MRIs, CT scans, etc.) will be scanned for the most suitable scenario. Since the AI will be able to classify common and uncommon patterns in certain images, it will become better and better at identifying diseases and other anomalies.

2. Detecting and classifying known features.

The large datasets that are formed with the cumulation from different sources can be overwhelming and difficult to analyze. Organization and classification of known features aids in better diagnosis. *The Joint Pathology Centre (JPC),* which is the pathology reference center for the United States federal government as well as a part of the US Defense Health Agency, selected **Huron's artificial intelligence-enabled** Lagotto™ image search engine to index and search JPC's growing digital image archive, unlocking the wealth of knowledge housed in the repository to enhance research and enable easier data sharing with researchers, diagnosticians, and educators. By connecting these rich datasets like pathology reports, treatment plans, patient outcomes, and even data from genomics, Lagotto sets the foundation for new applications, such as predictive algorithms for personalized treatment plans or improved drug discovery.[5]

3. Identifying unknowns.

A pathologist assisted by AI will be able to realize the presence of newer patterns or unexpected relationships that might not have existed before. This has the potential to help us arrive at new conclusions every time an AI algorithm searches through databases, biobanks, or electronic medical records.

A study by Hegde and colleagues in 2019 described Google's AI methodologies that helped to improve search results for similar features in digital images, irrespective of whether they had been annotated by trained pathologists or scientists. The experts who reviewed the digital slides marked them with their interpretations before feeding them into the database so that the AI algorithm can analyze and learn to differentiate cellular and tissue-based morphology from them. The algorithm named SMILY (Similar image search for histopathology) used datasets of unlabeled images to find morphologically similar images to recognize newer patterns to make more accurate predictions.[6]

4. Reducing errors

Since diagnosis in pathology often follows a path of repeated rejection of hypotheses until a final interpretation is derived, AI algorithms are able to rapidly and accurately sort through the various differential diagnoses and narrow down the most appropriate causative or prognostic factors for a particular disease. Robust algorithms may even be able to perform *"transfer learning,"* whereby the rationale used to diagnose a disease manifestation on one organ or tissue sample can be transferred or applied to another type of tissue sample. With the help of AI, applications not only can the WSI be analyzed automatically, but it can also be shared with or verified by experts globally, which ultimately reduces chances of errors and improves the accuracy of reports.

5. *Academic or professional training*

Lagotto™ is a patented, content-based image retrieval software that enables instant search for similar digital slides within an institution or a global data set and accesses the knowledge in corresponding diagnostic reports, patient outcomes, and metadata. With this software, users can find similar cases and read multiple pathology reports from subspecialty experts in real-time, providing a **"virtual peer review"** for pathologists, researchers, and educators.[7]

6. *Saving Time*

Pathologists who use AI systems report time-saving benefits during diagnosis, ensuring that they can spend more of their workdays on challenging cases and allow AI to take care of the labor-intensive, routine ones. In 2018, Google developed an AI algorithm *called Lymph Node Assistant (LYNA)* in order to report metastatic breast cancer on slides. In a study conducted by Steiner and colleagues, board-certified pathologists conducted a diagnostic simulation where the lymph nodes were reviewed for micrometastases of breast carcinoma cells in two phases, once with LYNA's help and once without. This laborious task was made easier with LYNA than without, as it cut the average slide review time in half. This also proves the potential of assistive technologies in reducing the burden of repetitive tasks for identification. The time and energy saved can be utilized by pathologists to focus on challenging diagnosis or clinical tasks.

The study also showed that pathologists using LYNA were more diagnostically accurate than either those who were unassisted or just the LYNA program when used alone, suggesting the ideal outcome was when the best of both the human mind and AI were used together.[8]

Evidence of Successful Applications of AI in Pathology

Applications in Microscopy

Despite the growth in AI research, the utilization of these tools in real practice is challenging due to prohibitors like the high cost of implementing the digitalization of sections using slides and scanners. To circumvent this, it was proposed to integrate AI directly into the microscope, i.e., the Augmented Reality Microscope (ARM), which overlays AI-based data points onto the microscopic view of the sample, relayed through the optical pathway in real-time, enabling seamless application of the algorithms into the microscopic workflow. The ARM can also be retrofitted into existing light microscopes using ready-made components, instead of investments in whole slide imaging technology. Currently, the program has been tried for breast and prostate cancers, but the potential applications are limitless. The ARM can provide visual feedback, like text, arrows, heat maps, or contours to help the pathologist narrow down on tumor-affected areas, helping to detect, quantify, and classify cancers rapidly and effectively.[9]

This helps to bring AI directly to the end-user, meeting them where they are most comfortable … at their microscopes. The pathologist has ready access to deep learning as it moves away from the computer lab and into the medical lab.

Applications in Onco-Pathology

In the past few years, precision oncology has advanced significantly and moved towards predictive assays that can enable the stratification and selection of patients for treatment appropriately. The complex processes that lead to cancer formation and progression due to divergence of transcriptional or signaling networks that in turn disrupt the function of biomarkers based on gene expression or protein formation generate unique morphological features in stained tissue specimens. The large amount of permutational data generated from this has led to an interest in AI systems to help with diagnosis by teaching neural networks to identify tumor versus normal areas in tissue samples through digital whole slide imaging so that it can consciously refine its analysis on new data supplied.[10]

Deep Learning and machine learning applications are trained to look for particular morphological features through the analysis of digital pictures obtained by whole slide imaging (WSI) and scanning. Today, with the availability of powerful processors, cloud-based computing, and strong IT infrastructures, a workflow based on *pixel-pipelines* can be developed to create prognostic or diagnostic algorithms based on machine learning.[11]

A study conducted by Nagpal and colleagues in 2019 used a Deep Learning (DL) AI system to assign Gleason scores automatically after processing whole slide images of tissue resected from radical prostatectomy. When compared to the scoring done by general pathologists, with both sets of results checked by an expert genito-urinary pathologist, it was observed that the DL approach had an accuracy of 0.7 in predicting the Gleason score, whereas the pathologists had a mean accuracy of 0.6. This method of using the AI algorithm improved diagnostic accuracy, especially where specialist expertise is unavailable.[12]

While modern approaches to the treatment of breast cancer require classification of patients and disease profiles in order to provide tailored therapy and predict survival, this stratification is based on the interpretation of tissue slides, mitotic counting in cells, and histological grading with biomarker status, which has been delegated to AI-based software applied on WSI, to relieve the pathologists from time-consuming and labor-intensive tasks, which may have varied results due to their inherent subjectivity.[13]

Research conducted by Shamai and colleagues in 2019 used AI algorithms and a deep learning system to assess hormonal or biomarker status from tissue microarrays in patients with breast cancer, which was predicted with 92% accuracy. This suggests that deep learning models can assist pathologists with the molecular profiling of oncology cases.[14]

Applications in Inflammatory Pathology

Neoplastic pathology has always taken center stage in most deep learning studies while overlooking its potential in inflammatory conditions. A study conducted in 2019 by Martin and colleagues investigated the use of DL algorithms developed by *Indica Labs*[15] for non-neoplastic gastric biopsies when compared to the gold standard diagnoses by independent pathologists. The resulting sensitivity/specificity parings of manual screening accuracy versus deep learning showed that the algorithm could identify H. pylori at 95.7% and 100%, which suggests that a convolutional neural network (CNN) has the potential to be a good screening and diagnostic tool for H. pylori gastritis. *Indica Labs* provided the evaluation of the WSI, quantitatively, using HALO AI for analysis of the digital images and *HALO Link* for data management and seamless collaboration.[16]

Applications in COVID-19

Due to the global pandemic in 2020, the discovery of the novel coronavirus meant that healthcare systems around the world had to find easy ways to assimilate knowledge about how the virus affects different organs and body functions in a timely manner, to help with treatment efforts as well as research towards an effective vaccine. An initiative launched in May 2020, spearheaded by the US Federal Government with the support of Indica Labs, for computational pathology software and OCTO for IT systems support[17], aimed to build an adequate dataset of information about COVID-19. Blood and tissue samples were taken from patients who were either diagnosed with or succumbed due to the virus. Whole slide images were prepared from various organs, including renal, hepatic, and cardio-pulmonary tissue samples.

The digital images were annotated by expert pathologists. The metadata was compiled in a cloud-based repository, which can be utilized as an educational resource and for research and clinical trials aimed at discovering preventive or therapeutic alternatives for COVID-19. The repository is now hosted by the National Institutes of Health in the United States. The electronic database is augmented software from *Indica Labs' HALO Link™*, enabling collaboration and secure methods to analyze and share images.

Conclusion

In order to benefit from the many advantages that AI brings to the table, a general change in mindset is essential as pathologists and other medical professionals need to understand that it is their partnership and experience that is vital to the integration of better technology.

In addition, outdated IT infrastructures, storage space limitations for software and hardware, network latency, and lack of interoperability due to outdated EHR interfaces are real and significant barriers to large-scale implementation. Regulations and evidence-based validation of the tools that are developed are also required to promote buy-in from the medical community.

It is also evident that in spite of a few hurdles, AI is already making headway in its applications to improve digital and surgical pathology workflows and result outcomes, contributing largely to rapid, automated diagnosis and access to timely therapeutic interventions. It has the potential to disrupt conventional molecular and genomic-based testing, which are the standards for predicting re-occurrence and outcomes of treatment.

From the patients' point of view, AI tools can enhance the patient experience through applications and mobile devices, giving them access to their electronic health records, radiology, and pathology reports, and images, in a background of known genomics (precise, accessible genetic testing) and other population-based health data.

References/Further Reading

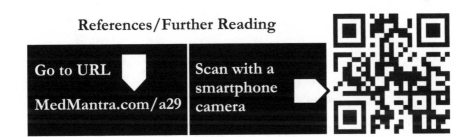

Go to URL
MedMantra.com/a29

Scan with a smartphone camera

CHAPTER THIRTEEN
SURGERY

In the coming decades, surgery done by humans will likely change dramatically, and the catalyst for the change will be the application of artificial intelligence in surgery, leading to faster and better patient care. Far from replacing surgical skills, AI-powered technology aims to ease the surgeon's burden and expand the possibilities of treatment.

The field of surgery in medicine itself has many specializations. Robotic surgery was introduced years ago to reduce the physical burden of practicing surgeons intra-operatively. AI, however, takes it a step further. The merging of AI applications with surgical robotics aims to reduce the cognitive burden as well by simplifying diagnosis and workflows with accurate and precise intra-operative maneuvers and the timely prediction of post-operative complications or morbidities.

Robotics in Surgery: The Foundation Laid

A surgeon's skill lies in finger dexterity and precise incisions. Their experience, obtained over years of training, is invaluable in the operating room. However, long and complicated surgical procedures are often physically demanding.

Surgical robots were invented and applied in the operating room, as they could execute multiple, repetitive surgical procedures precisely, under different levels of supervision, and could do so without fatigue. They also provided surgeons with a *"robotic wrist,"* which improved maneuvering and visualization within the surgical field. Ergonomics were also improved as kinematics were introduced, with large-scale human movements being scaled-down and converted into limited, complex, technical movements in the robotic hands. Robots could also avoid the very human tendency for unintended movements, hand tremors, or accidents that can have catastrophic results in surgery.

The very first robotic surgery, in 1985, was a simple neurosurgical procedure. A *stereotactic* brain biopsy was performed by a modified industrial robot called the *PUMA 560*. In 1994, *The Cyberknife* was invented, which used real-time image guidance, and a robotic arm to aim focused radiation beams for cancer treatment in patients who had inoperable or surgically complex tumors, using "stereotactic radiosurgery (SRS) as well as stereotactic body radiation therapy" (SBRT).

Since then, the area of surgical robotics has evolved rapidly to include *endoscopic* (the Zeus system in 1989 and the Da Vinci system in 2000), *bio-inspired* (the I-SNAKE and the CardioArm), and *micro-bot* models (capsule endoscopes like the PillCam). The development of *haptic feedback* technology, in which the robotic user interface could respond to touch, also introduced novel practical applications.[1]

However, the addition of AI to robotic surgery added a level of expertise that truly elevated the field and opened up a host of possibilities. The addition of different fields of AI like *Machine Learning (ML), Natural Language Processing (NLP), Artificial Neural Networks (ANN), and computer vision* has shown remarkable developments.

Applications of AI in Surgical Workflows and Robotics: The Future Built

While accuracy in robotics will greatly improve intra-operative surgical outcomes, the adoption of AI in pre-surgical and post-operative processes should also be considered in order to truly benefit patients going through surgery-based treatment modalities.

Machine Learning (ML) applied to electronic health records (EHR) has resulted in the design of a temporal prediction model that gives a data-based evaluation of patients for possible surgical site infections, based on an analysis of procedures, laboratory and radiological investigations, and patient symptoms, which gave remarkably accurate results as compared to traditional methods of diagnosis.[2]

Similarly, a Natural Language Processing (NLP) algorithm, the bag-of-words model, was applied to free text extracted from EHRs to diagnose the risk of anastomosis leakage after colorectal surgery, with 100% sensitivity and 72% specificity. This was done using surgeon notes about the operation, as well as predictive phrases that described patient symptoms or post-operative complaints.[3] Using Artificial Neural Networks (ANN) and Deep Learning, researchers were able to develop a clinical decision support system for surgeons evaluating a patient pre-operatively for an aortic vessel dilatation procedure, with 95.4% accuracy. Because the operation is very risky, the prediction of which patients are likely to develop complications or not survive the surgery is useful for reducing operational costs as well as post-procedure expenses due to expected morbidity. It gives patients the option for alternative treatments, knowing their predicted risk for surgical modalities, and helps to reduce undesirable post-procedure results.[4]

Computer vision algorithms can undertake an image-based analysis of patients' records that have surgical or diagnostic videos. Data absorbed from watching surgeons perform procedures, along with patient data from EHRs, can help to train machine learning systems to generate actionable information and even in identifying and predicting adverse events that may occur during or after surgical interventions in real time.

Fully Autonomous Systems: The Future Imagined

The first robot-assisted, trans-Atlantic telesurgery was conducted in 2001. It was termed "Operation Lindbergh" and involved gall bladder removal by a minimally invasive endoscopic procedure done while the patient was in an operating room at Strasbourg, France, while the surgeon operated a robotic console in New York, USA.[5]

To date, robotic surgery under teleguidance is an evolving prototype. Most systems under conceptualization do not leave decision-making to a robot, as they are performed with the surgeon's console within the operating room complex. Teleguided surgery is a more conventional option. A surgeon in the operating suite is at the local console, while an expert from another center not only visualizes but can even take over controls for certain crucial surgical steps. The implications of this technology in today's world are multi-fold. The doctor:patient ratio is drastically declining, leaving a dearth of specialty and super-specialty healthcare providers like surgeons. Therefore, it offers the ability for a clinically capable machine or robot to independently operate on patients in areas where human intervention is difficult, like those affected by natural disasters, endemic infections, or war zones, thereby maintaining both physician and patient safety, with good treatment outcomes.

In 2016, researchers initiated the *STAR trials (Smart Tissue Autonomous Robot)*, which used autonomous intestinal anastomosis procedures, employing only AI algorithms, with little or no human intervention at the controls. These trials gave AI its advent in surgical fields and provide a sneak peek at the future of truly intelligent machine applications in a skill-based, traditionally manual field in healthcare.[6,7]

Intraoperative applications of AI are, therefore, focused on guidance to facilitate improved visualization and localization during surgery. These are:

1. *Perception-based tools*: applications or software that trace the interactions between surgical tools and the environment, 3D reconstructions to show dynamic organ functions instead of static image displays, or instrument tracking and navigation.

2. *Localization and mapping of anatomical sites*: using *SLAM (Simultaneous Localization and Mapping) tools*[8], visual odometry and camera localization, endoscopic navigation, and augmented reality.

3. *System modeling and control tools*: using kinematics, machine learning from demonstrations through re-enforcement learning.

4. *Human-robot interaction tools:* using touchless manipulation or even intention understanding and prediction in the future.

In 2019, the *MicroSure* Robot, developed in the Netherlands for robotic microsurgery, used AI to suture small blood vessels in a patient with lymphoedema in order to reduce swelling.[9]

Early trials have been able to demonstrate that AI-assisted or controlled robotic surgery intraoperatively, or pre-operative and post-operative AI interventions, research-based guidance, or tools can help to reduce variations in clinical practice and procedures and thereby improve clinical outcomes. *Synaptive Medical recently tested its Modus V tool*, which is a fully automated, robotic digital microscope that can be used in operating rooms to visualize anatomical fields during the procedure.[10]

Proximie is a London-based web platform that allows doctors, especially surgeons, to communicate and collaborate through audio-video and augmented reality technology. Its AI-backed computer vision software enables surgeons to call upon data and images pertaining to the procedure and visualize it with unnatural clarity. "Proximie is now used by a third of all NHS hospitals, and the goal is to reach 40% penetration by the end of 2020" – Quote by Forbes magazine.[11]

Conclusion

Technology-based surgical practice can provide surgeons with the ability to improve care delivery. AI has the potential to collect and configure a vast database of surgical experience, similar to genomic databases and biobanks, to make clinical decision-making and complicated surgical techniques easier. Leveraging Big Data to create a "collective surgical consciousness" can lead to technology augmented and AI-controlled, real-time decision-making support, even leading to GPS-like guidance during an operation. Advanced AR and VR (Augmented Reality and Virtual Reality) systems can also step-up surgical training and teaching. If the technology is developed and implemented properly, AI can completely revolutionize the methods by which surgery is taught and applied, with the hope of a future primed to deliver optimum patient care.

References/Further Reading

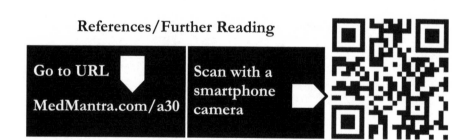

Go to URL
MedMantra.com/a30

Scan with a smartphone camera

CHAPTER FOURTEEN

ANESTHESIOLOGY

The field of anesthesiology is unique in medicine, as physicians involved in its practice must be equally involved with both their patients and other healthcare professionals, doctors, and nurses. Anesthesiologists must be familiar with drug metabolism, interactions, and timing while making critical decisions based on constantly changing patient variables and data inputs stemming from patient vitals and drug monitoring.

The introduction of Artificial Intelligence (AI) in healthcare aimed to make processes safer and more efficient for both physicians and patients. Anesthesia is no exception. Artificial Intelligence (AI) and Machine Learning (ML) can provide large quantities of highly accurate data, which can be processed efficiently, catering to patient-specific requirements.

AI has the potential to revolutionize the following areas in anesthesiology practice:

1. Depth of anesthesia monitoring

Distinguishing between awake and anesthetized states is one of the important problems in surgery. Vital sign parameters based on electroencephalogram (EEG) such as the Bispectral (BIS) - (Medtronic, USA) index have been used, as the EEG reflects brain activity to reveal information about different states of anesthesia that affect the brain, making it ideal for monitoring and predicting different depths of anesthesia (DoA).

Using recorded patient information as a data set for ML algorithms like LLE (Locally Linear Embedding) or ANN (Artificial Neural Networks), EEG signals can be classified into conscious and unconscious states for patients. Hence, researchers were able to develop a method for an EEG monitoring system that could assist anesthesiologists in accurately estimating the DoA during a surgery or procedure. Research conducted by Gu Y et al.[1] used ANN to analyze multiple EEG-based parameters like permutation entropy, Beta Ratio, and Synch Fast Flow to accurately distinguish between different patient states during propofol anesthesia. Similarly, Shalbaf et al. used data derived from EEG features to classify awake *versus* anesthetized patients during sevoflurane anesthesia with 92.91% accuracy.[2]

2. Control of anesthesia delivery

As the applications of BIS data derived from EEGs included being a key metric to measure the depth of anesthesia, researchers began to employ AI-based tools to achieve anesthetic control using BIS as a target measure. They also applied machine learning to regulate the delivery of anesthesia medications or mechanical ventilation. AI-dependent control systems that could automatically deliver drugs acting as neuromuscular blockades using rule-based hierarchy monitoring along with architecture framed with fuzzy logic control were used by Shieh et al., resulting in stable controller activity.[3]

Automated delivery of anesthesia by machine-based monitoring and weaning of mechanical ventilation has also been made possible through feedforward, feedback, or closed-loop systems.[4] Based on the patient's vital signs, the AI-based devices can automatically adjust DoA, which eliminates the need for the anesthesiologist to physically attend to the patient throughout a long surgical procedure. He may even be able to attend to multiple patients in adjacent OT rooms simultaneously, saving on manpower resources.

3. Event and risk prediction

The American Society of Anesthesiologists (ASA) has established a classification for the assessment of preoperative surgical patients for risk during surgery. Variations in interpretation have made uniform application of the ASA difficult, as often many variable patient factors must be considered, like the type of surgery, obesity, previous medical conditions, old age, etc. This leaves room for a considerable number of human errors. Hence, AI and deep learning algorithms were developed to guide physicians and surgeons through accurate allotment and interpretation of risk while using this grading system.

a. *Collection of patient data*

Anesthesia Touch™ is an AIMS (anesthesia information management and medication management system) for Android and iOS software that can enable automated and continuous charting of physiological data. Its user-friendly interface makes it comprehensive anesthesia documentation as well as a recorded patient electronic health record (EHR). Because AI-based monitoring devices can capture patient data automatically, the anesthesiologists need not write physical notes while attending to the patients.

Pharmacy Touch™ is a supplementary module that can automate documentation, thereby reducing drug errors, to support critical decisions in emergency situations at bedside care. This is integrated with **Synopsis Healthcare**, which specializes in the electronic preoperative assessment as well as anesthetic charting automation for the National Health Service (NHS) in the UK. **Synopsis iQ**[5] revolutionized the digital medication and monitoring role, making it clear and efficient. The platform reduces avoidable harmful events by improving consistency with interpretation. As a by-product, organizations can also reduce surgery or procedure cancellations with the efficient improvement of staff allocation and with increased patient turnover, decreasing unnecessary testing before procedures, and reducing malpractice risks.

b. Estimation of risk of difficult intubation

The preoperative identification of patients who exhibit signs of difficult intubation, through the use of automated, computerized assessments based on facial recognition software and trained AI algorithms, would reduce the incidence of adverse respiratory events due to anesthesia effects. A study conducted by Abdelaziz et al. used an ML algorithm called **Alex Difficult Laryngoscopy Software (ADLS)** along with the **Microsoft Visual Studio 2008** and **WEKA** (Waikato Environment for Knowledge Analysis) to identify intubations that were going to be difficult, with 76% accuracy.[6]

4. Ultrasound guidance

Artificial intelligence techniques have been used to assist the anesthetist in ultrasound-based procedures, most commonly undertaken to deliver medication. Hetherington et al. conducted a study based on a deep convolutional neural network (DCNN) to correctly identify vertebral levels to deliver epidural drugs. The algorithm discriminated between USG images of the lumbar vertebral spaces and bones with 80% accuracy. An augmented reality projection was displayed to show the anesthetist the vertebral level at the proposed puncture site.[7]

5. Pain management

Patient response to pain as well as to medication given to relieve pain can be estimated by AI-based neural networks to narrow down the specific drug and dosage required to lower pain scores, while titrating the amounts to prevent adverse reactions. This largely reduced trial and error methodologies, through predictive evidence-based algorithms, especially useful with post-operative pain, as well as patient-controlled chronic pain management.

Jose M et al. conducted a study using an analgesia monitor, the Analgesia Nociception Index (ANI) signal, to analyze the relationship between the ANI and drug titration made by the anesthesiologist, using machine learning techniques. The results, when cross-validated, can be used as an effective predictor for accurate dosages of pain management drugs.[8]

Procedure training by virtual reality

Simulation-based virtual reality training is rapidly finding its way into mainstream medical undergraduate as well as postgraduate courses. Traditional methods of training require immense time and resources from experienced and trained observers, which offers limited opportunities for learners to practice and hone skills for procedures. Virtual reality can provide repeated opportunities for the rehearsal of complex invasive procedures through simulation. The hardware required for VR training has also reduced in size, with the *Oculus* providing a cost-friendly and space-saving investment. Applied software like the *Anesthesia SimSTAT* is a screen-based training program developed by the American Society of Anesthesiologists and *CAE Healthcare*, which exposes learners to modeled pharmacology and live waveforms to help with anesthetic procedures for trauma, appendectomy, robotic surgery, and labor. The software is hosted on the Microsoft Azure platform, which also released its HoloLens 2, a wearable holographic computer, which allows for instinctual interactions with holograms, using AI algorithms to trace hand motions and eye gaze. This can train intensivists in casualty or ICU setups on emergency scenarios like cardiac arrest, strokes, head injuries, and bloodstream infections.[9]

AI will reduce errors and increase efficiency and perfection.

The goal of any AI-backed system is to efficiently decrease the cognitive load on physicians while taking over manual, time-consuming, and repetitive tasks so that the anesthesiologists can focus their attention on patients as well as on truly complicated cases that require skill-based interventions. At the end of the day, it is the patients who will benefit from more reliable and vigilant care delivery.

With the help of AI-based decision support systems in anesthesia, human errors and variances in interpretations will decrease, and efficiency will increase. AI-based anesthesia information management systems (AIMS) have smart monitoring systems that will ensure continuous monitoring and alarms during and after surgery to limit the effect of human errors or post-surgical complications.

AI will not replace professionals but will assist them.

While anesthesiology will reap benefits by using AI-based devices, machine learning is not a substitute for knowledge and judgment and cannot replace trained anesthesiologists. Manual skills and work-based experience are essential for carrying out emergency life-saving decisions. Most of the studies conducted in this arena deal with the augmentation of the anesthesiologist's workflow, decision-making, and clinical care, without the replacement of the physician's role, which combines both clinical knowledge and physical dexterity to undertake even routine activities like tracheal intubation, venous cannulation, and neural blockade, among others.

"Anesthesiologists enjoy a good mix of cognitive and dexterity-based labor, and given that AI will primarily result in the automation of cognitive work, it may be that our hands prevent full automation of the specialty," said Alexander and Josh, Baylor University Medical Centre.[10]

Over the last decade, machine learning and deep learning systems applied in anesthesiology are advancing in scope and number, with many exciting potential opportunities to bring the field into the future.

References/Further Reading

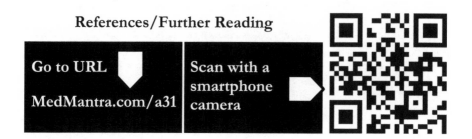

Go to URL

MedMantra.com/a31

Scan with a smartphone camera

CHAPTER FIFTEEN
PSYCHIATRY

Psychiatry is often thought to be reliant on human interaction. The psychiatrist sits with the patient or group of patients and listens to them speak about their troubles. From there, they address the situation with a diagnosis of a mental disorder or a similar mental health issue. Then, in a typical interaction, treatment with prescription drugs begins. Everything is done with a human psychiatrist at the helm—or is it? Similar to other medical fields, psychiatry is being quietly infiltrated by machines. The innovative technologies being born from advancements in artificial intelligence (AI) and machine learning are changing the delivery of psychotherapy that can be lifesaving for some patients.[1]

Mental Health Around the World

Approximately 792 million people have mental health problems globally, which translates to more than one in ten people. The National Institute of Mental Health (NIMH) has stated that 20% of adults in the United States, or 51.5 million people, suffer from at least one type of mental illness of various degrees of severity.[2] In Europe, around 83 million people have poor mental health, which is concerning because this includes people in some of the happiest countries in the world. Asia, too, has seen a sharp increase in people with mental illnesses. Aside from countries like Japan and South Korea having some of the highest rates of suicide in the world, Hong Kong has a population in which one in six people are afflicted by mental health woes. Unfortunately, due to the pandemic in 2020, this number is expected to grow in number and severity.

"There are huge unmet needs in psychiatry, with an acute shortage of psychiatrists and therapists in virtually every county in the U.S. and the shortage is even more dramatic in poorer countries," says Murali Doraiswamy, MD, professor of psychiatry and behavioral sciences and director of the neurocognitive disorders program at Duke University.

At the same time, there is a dearth of mental health professionals in the medical industry worldwide, and this shortage may lead to many people being unable to access psychiatric help when they need it.[3] Is this an area in which artificial intelligence (AI) can help? While many healthcare professionals, including psychiatrists, have different views when asked this question, recent developments suggest that AI may change the practice of psychiatric treatment modules for both physicians and patients.

Artificial Intelligence in Psychiatry at Present

The adoption of AI in psychiatry may be trickier than in other fields, like pathology or radiology, that deal with the recognition and correlation of images, patterns, or biomarkers to arrive at a diagnosis or formulate a treatment plan. Psychiatric symptoms cannot be tied down definitively to genetic codes, neuroimaging results, or brain activity patterns. The time and situational variances in brain functioning make it extremely difficult for technology to capture data.

The New Science of Human Behavior

In the realm of psychiatry, AI currently stands as a tool for assessment, with the initiation of a new branch called *"computational psychiatry."*

This field uses machine learning to increase data analysis and pull out the unknown factors beyond textbook mental disorders and illnesses or even much more unusual and extreme cases. In other words, AI makes it possible to mine psychiatric data and fabricate computer-aided experiments in which various personality traits and mental disorders are examined. There is also the potential to evaluate responses to medication in patients diagnosed with mental illnesses.

Use of AI in Mental Health Tools and Applications

1. mindLAMP

At the Beth Israel Deaconess Medical School, USA, the Division of Digital Psychiatry has developed an open-source project called *mindLAMP* ("Learn, Assess, Manage, and Prevent"), which uses a new technique called *digital phenotyping* through smartphone applications and sensors. The application gives clinicians and patients access to constantly updated real-time information regarding the patient's lived experience of mental illness, their true baseline, daily fluctuations, and reactions to life experiences, as well as responses to medications or treatment modules. The team has successfully secured their trial data and is using the app at their clinics. They have also managed to conduct surveys and cognitive tests through the software. With the application of machine learning algorithms to this data, researchers are looking to predict a patient's risk of serious mental illness or declining mental health status, and risk of relapse, so that adequate and timely interventions may be taken. The customizable application is currently available on both the Apple and Google app stores.[4]

2. Bi Affect

At the University of Illinois College of Medicine, the Departments of Psychiatry and Bioengineering created an application called Bi Affect, which has ingeniously analyzed an everyday feature in smartphones: the keyboard function. Studies have shown that patients suffering from bipolar disorder exhibit varying typing patterns depending on their change in moods. That is, during a manic episode, they tend to type faster, just like they would speak faster in person. Meanwhile, during a depressive episode, they tend to type shorter messages.[5]

Using this as a starting point, the team developed a deep learning algorithm (The *Deep Mood architecture*) which is applied to the keyboard metadata collected from the patient's smartphone. This captures and analyzes variations in typing speed, mistakes, pauses, backspace key use, etc., without collecting the matter that is being typed, in order to protect patient privacy. The analysis helped them to understand the correlation between mood swings and neurocognitive functioning.[6]

3. Cyberball Gaming Module

Cyberball is a computer game that measures social rejection. A subject controls one of the three players on the screen and believes that other people are controlling the remaining two, which are actually an AI-based algorithm. The researchers can then change the percentage of time the ball is passed to the human-controlled player to evoke feelings of rejection.

This type of algorithmic-based research has demonstrated how feelings of ostracism, social exclusion, or rejection may be different when comparing people with or without borderline personality disorders.[7]

4. Instagram Learning

They say a picture is worth a thousand words. Harvard University and the University of Vermont researchers believe this to be true, and so they took to Instagram with machine learning to seek out a means of improving depression screening. The AI diagnosed depression accurately in the trial participants, using photo metadata, color analysis, and algorithm-based face detection, and managed to outperform health practitioners' unassisted diagnostic success rate.[8]

5. Chat Bots

a. Tess by X2AI

Created by X2AI, Tess is AI software that asks all the questions people need to hear via text messages. The software can even administer psychotherapy to those afflicted with depression and emotional instability. According to X2AI's CEO and co-founder, Michiel Rauws, Tess is a psychological artificial intelligence that uses natural language processing to understand what the user is actually talking about, to pick up on human expressions like, "I don't want to wake up anymore in the morning." Then it delivers coping strategies or immediate aids for the situation.[9]

b. Woebot

Woebot is a digital cognitive behavioral therapist, accessible through smartphone mobile apps. The inbuilt AI algorithm is capable of having conversations with users to track their moods through videos and word games. After analysis, it devises recommended treatments based on scores and conversations. For instance, Woebot will ask, "How are you feeling?" and then proceed to emulate a face-to-face discussion with an actual human psychiatrist.[10]

6. IBM Research Through Watson

You might have recently read about ongoing studies that are looking into how people with various mental illnesses and problems verbalize themselves differently from others. The chances are that some of the latest research was assisted by AI. IBM has been collecting transcripts and audio clips from psychiatric interviews and paired this data with its algorithms, like Watson, to find patterns in speech. The hope is that having AI learn about these patterns can help with predicting and monitoring schizophrenia, mania, depression, and psychosis. Presently, IBM's AI needs to hear only about 300 words from a client before it detects the probability of psychosis, thus aiding in faster diagnosis and treatment.

Predictive Power

Researchers at Stanford's Center for Precision Mental Health and Wellness used an AI-based algorithm to interpret the brainwave patterns of people diagnosed with depression, before and after they were given medications for their symptoms, in order to predict which symptoms would change with the treatment given. In a mammoth task, individual patient symptoms were combined with individual electroencephalography (EEG) results at different points during the treatment. It was concluded that the algorithm could successfully identify patients with a higher risk of poor prognoses, such as suicidal tendencies, which may have otherwise been missed due to the subjective nature of traditional examinations. The validation of these processes, as well as large-scale implementation in resource-poor countries, may delay the adoption of the technology.[11]

Benefits of AI in Psychiatry

Using artificial intelligence as part of a psychiatric evaluation has a host of benefits. Looking briefly at other medical fields where AI is being integrated, there have been reports of streamlined workflow, earlier detection and treatment of diseases like cancer, and enhanced detection of abnormalities in radiology data (MRIs, CT scans, etc.). The advantages of AI to psychiatry would be as follows:

1. **Easy accessibility**

   One of the biggest hindrances in the medical field for both healthcare professionals and patients is the lack of accessibility. According to studies, 56.4% of adults and over 60% of adolescents suffering from mental illness do not receive treatment. There is a global drought of psychiatric support systems.[12]

   AI, however, could be a starting point for bringing psychiatric care to those who need it the most. Chatbots like *Tess* and *Woebot* can provide rudimentary consultations, while *online platforms like Ginger.io*[13,14], a partnership of machine learning and a clinical network, can provide suggestions or real-time support to users as well as an array of treatments through video-based therapy and psychiatry sessions.

2. **Faster detection**

   Traditional psychiatric care was dependent on the patient's personal observations (or lack thereof) to make inferences on the issue, as well as professional observations and reporting. However, with AI created by IBM's Computational Psychiatry and Neuroimaging group, and research by universities and other technological startups, AI is now able to use methods like natural language processing (NLP) to use a patient's speech to predict mental illness or the onset of psychosis.[15]

3. **Using AI for research-based tools to identify vulnerable populations**

   A team of MIT and Harvard University researchers used natural language processing algorithms to identify similarities in social media posts and thereby identify groups of people who expressed anxiety or isolation, referred to substance abuse, etc., during the last year. The number of people had significantly increased as compared to similar studies conducted in 2018 and 2019. This kind of analysis could aid in the identification of population groups that are most vulnerable to adverse mental health effects rooted in major events like the Covid-19 pandemic, political effects, or natural disasters.

If the algorithms were applied in real time to social media posts, they could be used to immediately offer online resources, like guiding people to online support groups, highlighting information on how to find mental health treatment, or even facilitating contact with a suicide hotline.[16]

Conclusion

AI and psychiatry can form a formidable partnership in the fight against mental illness and personality disorders. With digitization and automation of selected tasks, such as asking questionnaires, detecting various speech patterns, and thought processes, AI can aid those who need it most and also help psychiatrists detect problems faster than ever before. A multidisciplinary approach toward establishing a rigorous framework to evaluate new studies that deal with the applications of AI algorithms should be established for rapid and transparent validation. Though AI still has its limitations, the potential for the technology to improve the diagnosis and the delivery of mental health care is undeniable.

References/Further Reading

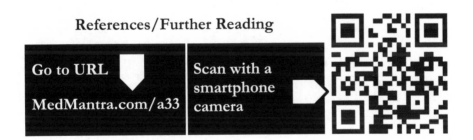

Go to URL
MedMantra.com/a33

Scan with a smartphone camera

CHAPTER SIXTEEN
CARDIOLOGY

Cardiology and technology have always been intertwined. Without electrocardiograms, echocardiograms, cardiac catheterization, and similar modalities, cardiology would not exist as it does today. However, to meet the growing population of people with cardiac problems and ailments, cardiologists are finding that they need the help of computers so that they can become more efficient and effective in their line of work. When artificial intelligence arrived as a possible solution, it seemed like science fiction, restricted to far-fetched research projects. However, the rapid pace at which AI methods have progressed has resulted in the widespread adoption of these technologies, with many gaining market clearances from the FDA (U.S. Food and Drug Administration). With the incorporation of machine learning, deep learning, and other AI systems into healthcare, one may already be using and experiencing an AI system or algorithm for themselves, without even realizing it.

But just how far have AI and machine learning come in terms of cardiology? Moreover, what future developments can we hope to see within our lifetimes? In the field of cardiology, the future is now!

The State of Artificial Intelligence in Cardiology

Even though technology and medicine are gradually becoming dependent on one another, the idea of AI as an engineering tool for creating innovations in cardiovascular medicine has yet to truly catch on. However, progress is being made in these major areas:

1. Prediction of risk and outcomes

2. Imaging and diagnostics

3. Clinical decision support (CDS) after thorough validation

Here is a look at the latest innovations that came about due to the integration of AI with cardiology.

1. Prediction of Risks and Outcomes

Machine learning through AI is a robust and innovative tool that can help with cardiovascular risk stratification by incorporating nontraditional or unknown risk factors, thereby helping with preventive measures rather than curative.

a. *Microsoft's Healthcare Next Initiative*

Around March 2017, Microsoft launched the *Microsoft Intelligent Network for Eyecare (MINE)* in places like Australia, Brazil, India, and the US. MINE was renamed the AI Network for Healthcare because, soon after its launch, Microsoft partnered with Apollo Hospitals, one of the largest healthcare providers in India. The project became a part of *Microsoft's Healthcare Next Initiative*. The goal was to use AI to develop treatment guidelines and proven clinical algorithms in cardiology. The *National Clinical Coordination Committee (NCCC)* was also set up soon after, with the aim of constructing an India-specific heart risk score, in order to predict cardiovascular ailments for the Indian demographic, as opposed to using tools based on data derived from Western studies.

The corporate VP of Microsoft AI and Research, Peter Lee, stated, "By working side by side with the healthcare industry's most pioneering players, we are bringing Microsoft's capabilities in ground-breaking research and product development to help healthcare providers, biotech companies, and organizations around the world use artificial intelligence and the cloud to innovate".[1]

On analyzing a large database of patients with heart disease, the team was able to narrow down 21 risk factors that can predict the occurrence of cardiovascular events, which could change the way preventive health checks are done, as well as provide insight to physicians with early diagnosis and effective treatment plans.

Further, the team is working on an *AI-powered Cardio API platform* that could potentially predict a patient's heart risk score just by providing a detailed history, without investigations if not required, thereby streamlining operations. With an IT giant like Microsoft getting into biomedical technologies, one can anticipate many remarkable inventions.[2]

177

b. Google's Verily Software

Google's health-tech subsidiary **Verily** determined that it's AI algorithms could assess a person's risk of developing heart disease by reviewing scans from the back of a patient's eye, i.e., through a retinal scan. The algorithms could determine the patient's age, smoking habits, and blood pressure from the images, thereby predicting the individual's risk of cardiovascular disease, with almost 70% accuracy.[3]

c. Wearable Sensors

The application of remote patient monitoring in the evaluation of an individual's health has empowered patients to take control of their well-being. Smart bands or watches have been upgraded with ECG monitors that can pick up wave abnormalities and transmit the data in real time to treating physicians. Patient-generated data, when analyzed, can help create a database for future risk predictions incorporating a more diverse population group. A study conducted by **Tison and colleagues** attempted to passively detect atrial fibrillation using ECG reports generated from commercially available smartwatches, coupled with a deep neural network.[4]

At the **University of Nottingham in the UK,** researchers had AI teach itself, through machine learning, to find patterns in data and predict which patients would have a heart attack within ten years. The AI system scanned more than 300,000 patient records to make these predictions. At the end of the study, the researchers found that the AI algorithms predicted heart attacks with greater accuracy than the assessments created by the American College of Cardiology / American Heart Association.[5]

2. Imaging and Diagnostics

a. Arterys MICA in Cardiac MRI

One name that both radiologists and cardiologists are most likely familiar with by now is **Arterys Medical Imaging Cloud AI (Arterys MICA)**, which is an online medical imaging analytics program powered by AI. The system combines both cloud supercomputing and accelerated workflow to deliver results. The Cardio-based AI system has functions like 2D and 4D Flow blood imaging and 3D Cine for ventricular volumes. The algorithm is applied rapidly to perfusion datasets and signal intensity graphs from *cardiac MRI software* to deliver accurate, semi-quantitative segmental analysis that enables faster patient examinations by up to 30%, saving at least 25 minutes per LV/RV (left ventricle/right ventricle) function segmentation.

Presently, Arterys is partnered with Siemens Healthineers and GE ViosWorks. Interestingly, Siemens Healthineers is working alongside GE and IBM Watson to enhance medical imaging.[6]

b. *Caption Health in Echocardiography*

Caption Health (originally Bay Labs Inc.) is a US-based AI company devoted to using deep learning to help healthcare professionals in developing countries. The company brought deep learning to Kenya to help doctors identify rheumatic heart disease (RHD) and congenital heart disease. It previously tested its algorithms at the Minneapolis Heart Institute and Allina Health, Northwestern Medicine, Duke University School of Medicine, and cardiologists at Stanford University, to help cardiologists accurately interpret 2D echo studies.[7] The algorithm can automatically calculate ejection fractions while scanning from three cardiac views at the point of care, providing a quick visual assessment.[8]

c. *Convolutional Neural Networks*

In 2020, *Kusunose and colleagues*[9] used convolutional neural networks (CNN) to identify regional wall motion abnormalities in the cardiac musculature, from echo-cardiographic images, which demonstrated that the deep learning algorithm was able to diagnose the abnormalities as accurately as cardiologists or sonographers during the trial. This created the possibility of using CNN for automated diagnosis in echocardiography

Rima Arnaout[10], a cardiologist and assistant professor at UC San Francisco, created a deep learning CNN that applied an algorithm to categorize cardiac ultrasounds and detect congenital heart disease from fetal ultrasounds according to the type of view, with 92% accuracy as compared to 79% attained by human experts.

d. Analytics 4 Life

The Toronto-based company Analytics 4 Life has created the Corvista system, which is a new cardiac diagnostic platform. It is a point-of-care system that collects signals transmitted by the heart through leads while the patient is at rest. It is usually a three-minute recording that collects 10 million data points. This data is uploaded to the system's secure cloud database to create a three-dimensional image of the heart. AI-based machine learning algorithms are performed on the patient's data and help to determine the presence of cardiovascular disease through Phase Space Tomography. The test results are sent to clinicians immediately after the procedure for rapid intervention in cases of coronary artery disease, pulmonary hypertension, or heart failure. The device is being used in Canadian hospitals as a non-invasive diagnostic application.[11]

3. Clinical Decision Support

Point-of-care clinical decision-making tools are required as patient management becomes increasingly complex with the introduction of a variety of investigation and treatment options. Evidence-based guidelines are required to bring about good results, especially with the incredible range of electronic data available. Analysis of this data to arrive at actionable conclusions and recommendations has been a challenge for cardiologists thus far.

With the use of structured data sets like laboratory investigation reports, patient demographic information, and electrocardiography and physiology reports, machine learning algorithms have been able to accelerate diagnosis and predict risks and disease outcomes. With the addition of clinical narratives, through patient electronic health records (EHR), the data sets become augmented and complete, leading to better analysis. Extrapolating this information from EHRs was a challenge that was adequately resolved through the application of *natural language processing (NLP) algorithms* that add input to clinical decision support systems, making them more robust and accurate.

Weissler E and colleagues[12] applied trained NLP algorithms to patients' electronic health data in order to accurately diagnose peripheral artery disease, thereby leading to better interventions for patient care, while automatically estimating the prognosis. The Mayo Clinic has used data-empowered NLP software like *MEd Tagger*, which is an Open Health Natural Language Processing Consortium, for information extraction.[13]

Conclusion: The Future Is in the Research

Artificial intelligence and machine learning have led to a plethora of technological advancements in the field of cardiology. The studies that have recently been published bolster the already proven usefulness of AI systems. Yet, the future lies within the research.

Presently, many AI systems are based on imaging, reducing workload, and increasing both the productivity and the efficiency of medical field professionals. The enhancement of cardiac and other medical images provides doctors and surgeons with a sharper eye. AI is helping professionals make clearer, more informed decisions, leading to better patient outcomes with reduced mortality and morbidity rates. The challenge will be the adoption and implementation of this software in widespread clinical environments, when medical professionals realize that the real power of AI is to improve clinical efficacy by enhancing the clinician-patient interface, instead of replacing it. AI will become an indispensable partner in healthcare, especially when we get to the heart of the matter.

References/Further Reading

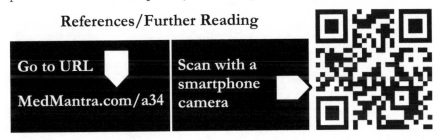

Go to URL
MedMantra.com/a34

Scan with a smartphone camera

CHAPTER SEVENTEEN

PHARMACY

In 2022, the pharmaceutical industry is thriving in ways it always has. Scientific discoveries influence the creation or reconstruction of certain medications, and new methods to quell epidemics, diseases, and other ailments affecting society are born. Yet, as new technologies beyond pharmacology are being introduced, the idea of what the "pharmacy" is and how it can evolve to better serve the future comes into question. How will advancements like artificial intelligence (AI) and machine learning (ML) alter the course of pharmacology and pharmaceutical company practices? As it turns out, AI is already having an impact on many realms of the healthcare system; pharmacy included.[1]

In fact, AI was woven into pharmacy more in 2020 than ever before. According to one of the recent trending topics, artificial intelligence has gained the attention of pharmaceutical giants like Johnson & Johnson, Merck, and GlaxoSmithKline. Each company has invested heavily in machine learning, hoping that AI will build "prediction models for potentially promising compounds." Right now, it takes up to 15 years for a new drug to be produced, starting from the moment of discovery to the proper execution—and that means over US$1 billion spent on the manufacturing and testing of a single drug type.

The hope is that AI will be able to manufacture new, more effective drugs with more celerity and for less production costs.

Current State of Artificial Intelligence in Pharmacy

But while investments from big enterprises is one step towards an AI-enriched future, what is happening between artificial intelligence and the pharmaceutical field presently?

The usefulness of AI is not solely limited to approximations and finding patterns. Presently, there are programs being developed that allow AI to detect specific symptoms or anomalies, add to the diagnostic process, develop treatment protocols, aid in medicine manufacturing, as well as monitoring and caring for patients. The main purpose of all these programs and deep learning algorithms is to lessen the burden on the human professionals and streamline the workload.

We see AI being incorporated into every facet of healthcare, ranging from

- Computers – faster data collection, better data processing

- Data recording in healthcare devices

- Creation of gene databases and pharmacogenomics

- Faster adoption of electronic health records and databases

- Systems with natural language processing capabilities to automate certain processes in the healthcare field.

What that means for pharmacies is that AI has already begun supporting researchers with making decisions about existing medications and drugs and various treatments. AI is also to be used to predict where epidemics may occur by having it learn the history of outbreaks through records and other media sources. However, it is safe to say that artificial intelligence and deep machine learning can be taken even further.

Future Hopes for AI and Pharmacy

Though much of the technology that will become more ubiquitous in the future is already under progressive development, the anticipation is that the integration of AI into the pharmacy and other fields in healthcare will expand rapidly by 2030.

AI and ML

Algorithms that can "learn" will play an integral role in the future, especially during drug development. Researchers will have access to a wealth of collected scientific data to work with, thanks to the efforts of AI gathering information from all over the world. Thus, research can be conducted quicker, aiding in the formation of new knowledge.

Benevolent Bio and its customized AI is the perfect example of this. Jackie Hunter of Benevolent Bio states, "The AI we've developed—embodied in the company's Judgement Correlation System (JACS)--is able to review billions of sentences and paragraphs from millions of scientific research papers and abstracts."

In other words, this system called JACS finds links in data and names it "known facts" about a specific condition or disease. Then these known facts are compiled, and further patterns or connections are made. The end result is that the JACS generates hundreds of hypotheses based on the criteria inputted by the scientists. Once the hypotheses are created, researchers discuss the most plausible and start testing the top 5 in the lab.

Streamlined workflow and a greater perspective of how and why ailments begin are a few of the major benefits of AI, and it's only to become more helpful in the future.

Personalized Pharmacy

In current times, a visit to the pharmacy means dealing with long lines, exorbitant prices, and no time to consult with the professionals behind the counter. One hope for AI in the future is to set up booths that allow for the patient to receive proactive care. For example, a system being utilized now is "Intouch Health," a telehealth network in remote locations of the US. Anyone using the system can access consultations for various conditions.

Additionally, AI and ML will increase the availability of personalized therapies. With the dissemination of cloud-based technologies and digitized healthcare systems, pharmacies will be able to receive information from primary healthcare providers and hospitals on-demand. This can even lead to advancements like the already FDA-approved epilepsy drug called Spritam that's made using 3D printers. The drug is layered, making it faster to dissolve than regular epilepsy drugs. Now imagine if pharmacies all had 3D printers to distribute necessary medication to those in need with the push of a button.

AI programs will be integrated into the electronic medical records, which will raise an immediate alarm if a physician tries to prescribe a medicine which the patient is allergic to or is incompatible with a medicine which the patient is already taking. AI programs will rapidly calculate the minimum possible but most effective dose of medicines after considering all patient-specific factors like body weight, biochemical results, other health conditions, etc.

That's the future of preventative healthcare. That's the future of pharmacy.

Conclusion

When it comes to a blending of artificial intelligence and pharmacy, there already are connections that have been made, even within the pharmacy management system, such as drug utilization data and clinical decision opinion screenings. AI is in the workflow, too. Thus, we are beginning to see a world where AI is shifting the focus away from the more mechanical side of pharmacy, such as the data collection and manufacturing of new drugs, and to the more human elements, like collaborating with other countries, optimizing health and wellness, and preventing catastrophic epidemics from spreading in the future. AI is already a major component of pharmacy, so it now comes down to accepting the advantages and implementing new methods of use.

References/Further Reading

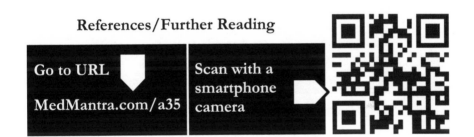

Go to URL
MedMantra.com/a35

Scan with a smartphone camera

CHAPTER EIGHTEEN
DERMATOLOGY

Even though artificial intelligence applications are in the early stages of development in the healthcare sector, their current abilities are broad, and they are already improving the general state of healthcare.[1]

Furthermore, some centers in the United States have locally developed systems that give pop-up notifications to alert doctors when a specific drug or medication may not work with a patient based on some concrete reasons like genetic traits.[1]

These apps can also give physicians practical reasons; their major areas of specialization are skin image analysis and personalized skincare treatment.

Regarding Skin Image Analysis, AI-based dermatology companies are creating applications and devices using computer learning and machine learning to analyze photos to predict and prevent skin diseases from occurring.

Content-Based Image Retriever

Apart from predictive analytics and data management, artificial intelligence is used in the area of dermatology via the use of CBIR- content-based image retriever. The CBIR functions are culled from the skin image analysis.

DermEngine's Visual Search and Skin Vision are perfect examples of such dermatology apps. This intelligent dermatology software focuses on identifying skin cancer images and gives the medical professional visually similar pictures with the top diagnosis and the risk of malignancy of these past cases.

DermEngine's Visual Search

It uses deep learning and image processing technologies to aid medical experts in their clinical decisions, and it is also beneficial in training or to new physicians who want to specialize in skin cancer.

SkinVision

SkinVision is built solely to use machine vision to check for skin lesions for risk of cancer through photosynthesis.

It was founded in 2011 in the Netherlands; this app is sophisticatedly trained on a database of over one million images of skin lesions; the algorithm learns to recognize particular features like shape, color, and which one may indicate a higher risk of melanoma.

Skin10

Skin10 is yet another app developed to help dermatologists diagnose skin conditions; its algorithm is built on an extensive database of skin conditions, although the sources of database images are unclear.

How does it work?

All that the patients have to do is to download the Skin10 app and sign up for Skin10's network.

Secondly, users take pictures of the region of their body where they wish to analyze. However, the system can also process the entire body parts, and such scans can be integrated by using an overlay feature in the app camera. Skin10 can detect skin conditions like solar lentigo, lipoma, and malignant melanoma.

For the good of humanity

Artificial intelligence is making work easier for dermatologists; apart from skin image analysis, AI is also proving to be valuable in the area of personalized skincare treatments. Companies are building recommendation engines to personalize skincare treatment recommendations to user skin type.[1]

On a broad scale, access to high-quality data and incompatibilities between different electronic medical record databases are current challenges. However, AI-based Dermatology Company is an example of the perfect start-up company- cited by Eric Schmidt (Chairman of Alphabet Inc., the parent company of Google). Using crowd-sourced input from dermatologists, he imagined machine learning and deployed it via smartphone technology, which can create a highly accurate artificial intelligence diagnosis tool.[1]

Furthermore, an obvious concern is a possibility that AI may infringe on physicians' practice. The boundary between making clinical decisions and making recommendations remains to be drawn.

Nevertheless, at this development stage of AI in dermatology, we still cannot rely solely on a computer to tell us what to do; a medical judgment that involves a conversation with a patient is best left to the treating physician.[1]

References/Further Reading

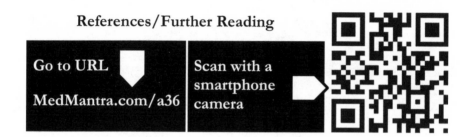

Go to URL

MedMantra.com/a36

Scan with a smartphone camera

CHAPTER NINETEEN
DENTISTRY

Over the course of history, we have come to understand that communities always adopt the right and essential technology. One thing we are sure about is that artificial intelligence is positively changing the healthcare industry, including dentistry—and doing so faster than anyone could imagine.

This aspect of healthcare is not afraid or skeptical about implementing some of these new technologies. From management software to 3D printing to digital radiographs, dentists are the early adopters of these revolutionary inventions. Moreover, the next evolution of dental technology and its rapid adoption will be made possible through artificial intelligence-based products.

The Rise of AI-Based Technology in Dentistry

With the help of AI-based applications, it is now possible to detect the efficacy of various treatment methods considering anatomical conditions and distinct symptoms, using artificial intelligence and large datasets of diagnostic results, treatments, and outcomes. It is essential given the assortment of new dental techniques, materials, and technologies, which are introduced annually.

Applications of Artificial Intelligence in Different Fields of Dentistry

The last decade was considered the decade of vital achievements in the field of artificial intelligence. There are various practical applications of AI-based systems in dentistry:

1. **Artificial intelligence in patient management**

    An AI-based virtual dental assistant can perform different patient management tasks in a dental practice with more accuracy and less error. In departments such as oral pathology, oral medicine, and radiology, it can be used to manage patient appointments as well as to assist in diagnosis or to plan subsequent treatments.[1] It also works by notifying the dentist about the patient's complete dental and medical history, including details about alcohol consumption, smoking and tobacco use, oral hygiene habits, and food and other dietary habits.[2] Thus, a virtual database for each patient is developed to aid the dentist in prompt diagnosis and subsequent treatment of complex dental diseases.[1,2]

2. Artificial intelligence in the diagnosis and treatment of different dental problems

AI-based trained neural networks can be used to diagnose complex dental diseases having multifactorial etiology. This is a precious gift that artificial intelligence has given to clinical dental practice, as a correct diagnosis is a strong foundation for proper treatment. An example of this is the recurrent aphthous ulcer, which is a condition without a specific cause or with multifactorial etiology; trained neural networks can diagnose it based on the recurrence of the lesion and the exclusion of other factors.[3] AI can also precisely prognosticate a predisposition to oral cancer genes and tooth surface loss for a large population by using genetic algorithms of the oral lesions as well as the genetic algorithms of unerupted canines or premolars.[4]

3. Artificial intelligence in prosthetic dentistry

To render perfect prostheses for patients, various influencing factors such as esthetics, anthropological calculations, facial measurements, and patient preferences have been integrated by an AI-based system (RaPiD) for successful use in prosthetic dentistry. These AI-based systems integrate computer-aided manufacturing (CAM), knowledge-based systems, and computer-aided design (CAD) as a unifying medium for successful dental restoration with great accuracy.[5] CAD/CAM techniques are used in the manufacturing of inlays, onlays, crowns, and bridges.[6] AI plays a main role in the identification of the type of bone as well as the cortical thickness in order to make precise surgical guides for the placement of implants. It has replaced the time-consuming conventional methods of routine casting, thereby reducing the required time as well as errors.

4. Artificial intelligence in oral and maxillofacial surgery

AI software programs can help in the planning of oral and maxillofacial surgeries by providing the smallest details regarding vital structures around the craniofacial region in order to preserve them during the surgical procedures.[7] The extraordinary application of artificial intelligence in this field is the introduction of robotic surgery (in which human intelligence and human body motion are simulated). Removal of tumors and foreign bodies, oral implant surgery, biopsy, and temporomandibular joint surgeries are some common successful applications of AI-guided oral and maxillofacial surgeries.[8]

5. Artificial intelligence in orthodontics

AI-driven customized orthodontic diagnostics and treatments have revolutionized the field of orthodontic dentistry. AI algorithms and statistical analysis can be used in multiple orthodontics processes, from precise diagnosis to treatment planning and even to follow-up prognostic monitoring. AI-based intraoral 3D scanners and cameras can analyze different radiographs and photographs of relevant craniofacial and dental regions and aid in diagnosis as well as treatment planning.[9] From these photographs and radiographs, a data-driven algorithm can be developed. Final treatment outcomes, tooth movement, and pressure points for those specific teeth can be predicted by applying these algorithms and statistical analysis. Thus, AI-driven customized orthodontic treatment not only provides accurate treatment but also minimizes the chances of errors while reducing the treatment time.[10]

6. Artificial intelligence in radiology

AI-integrated imaging scans such as MRI and cone-beam CT may assess minor changes from normal that remain hidden to the human eye, e.g., artificial neural networks (ANNs) can localize minor apical foramen by magnifying the radiographs and aiding in the diagnosis of proximal caries.

In the last 5-10 years, image recognition in the radiology practice by using AI-based systems has shifted from science fiction to reality. AI provides an additional advantage in craniofacial imaging due to the distinctive ability of deep learning to identify minor deviations. AI algorithms can detect maxillary sinusitis on panoramic radiographs, and Sjogren syndrome on CT scans at early stages in order to prevent severe complications in the future.[11]

7. Artificial intelligence in periodontics

By using various radiographs and photographs, deep learning analysis tools can help in the diagnosis and treatment planning of complex periodontal diseases. AI can be used in the early detection of periodontal variations, bone loss, and variations in bone density, which helps in early intervention in dental implant systems.[12]

Convolutional neural networks can successfully detect periodontitis of premolars and molars. AI can also analyze the immune response profile of the patients and effectively categorize these patients into aggressive and chronic periodontitis. Thus, AI can guide dental professionals in optimum treatment protocols.[13]

8. Use of genetic algorithms to optimize dental implant systems

AI-based genetic algorithms work based on the "survival of the fittest" principle. Genetic algorithms can be used to optimize dental implant systems and determine the lifespan of restorative materials so that they can be chosen wisely. These algorithms can be applied to improve tooth color matching in prosthodontics. Statistical analysis based on genetic algorithms can predict dental caries at the initial stages to avoid future dental decay.[14] AI-driven genetic algorithms based on CAM/CAD can be used in the reconstruction of missing parts of the tooth and to maintain the overall smoothness of the reconstructed tooth surface.

9. Clinical decision support system in dentistry

A clinical decision support system (CDSS) based on inbuilt clinical knowledge supports dental professionals in making clinical decisions about the diagnosis, treatment, prognosis, and prevention of various dental problems. For example, when a patient with a toothache visits a dentist, the CDSS immediately analyzes all the relevant data through a short questionnaire filled out by the patient and automatically suggests a treatment plan.[15]

10. Artificial intelligence in endodontic dentistry

ANNs can be used to detect vertical root fractures as well as to localize minor apical foramen (*small* accessory canals at the tip or *apex* of some teeth roots) in the field of endodontic dentistry. ANNs can enhance the success of root canal treatment by increasing the accuracy of working length determination by up to 96%, which is greater than the accuracy attained by a professional endodontist.[16]

11. Artificial intelligence in forensic odontology

ANNs can be used to determine gender or age by using different dental parameters with minimal errors.[16] Automated techniques based on ANNs can be used effectively in forensic odontology to identify victims of child abuse, sexual assault, crimes, mass calamities, and other legal issues.

12. Artificial intelligence in pediatric dentistry

AI-driven CAD restorative design and manufacturing can be used in pediatric restorative dentistry to achieve great results in terms of time required and esthetics. The sizes of interrupted premolars and canines can be predicted during the mixed dentition period by using artificial neural networks.[17]

13. Prediction of dental problems by using ANN predictive models

ANN predictive models based on the association between tooth pain and daily brushing frequency, brush time, toothbrush replacement patterns, and other factors such as diet and exercise can effectively predict toothaches. ANN models can also be used to predict the expected timelines for dental extraction in orthodontic dentistry. Data mining analysis can determine the lifespan of restorative materials to choose them intelligently for suitable cases.

14. Artificial intelligence in community dentistry

AI-driven models can be used in community dentistry, including diagnostic recommendations for various dental problems, standard dental therapy protocols, personalized medicine, and even the prediction of epidemiological disease spread from a global perspective.

AI-based oral health mobile apps can track and educate a person about monitoring his/her dental health through an AI-based scanner in the app and regularly remind users about oral hygiene.[17]

15. **Artificial intelligence in craniofacial cancer prediction**

Using CT scan images, convolutional neural networks (CNNs) can predict areas in the head and neck with a high risk of cancer. Genetic programming (GP) can be used in the oral cancer prognosis by statistical analysis of different genetic factors.[18] Artificial neural networks (ANNs) can be used in the identification and grading of high-risk craniofacial cancer patients to plan a treatment regime accordingly.

Meet Some of the New Technologies

Orthy

Orthy was founded in 2016 by Patrick Y Lee. This AI-based tech claims to have the right elements to be the future of cosmetic dentistry with regard to invisible aligners. Without any doubt, Orthy has improved dental treatment by making aligner treatments more convenient and affordable. The app is built to predict the future smile of the patient after treatment. Users tap to request their snapshot for a 30-minute appointment with a dentist in the area. Then they get scanned and get X-rays done. If the patient is a good fit, in 24 hours, he or she can see the results in terms of his or her future smile.

Dentistry.AI

This is yet another benefit of artificial intelligence in dentistry. The digital health app is a cloud-based AI technology that physicians can use to detect dental caries on x-rays (bitewings).

The United States FDA has approved the caries detection software (by Dentistry.AI) for clinical use but as an investigational device. Moreover, Dentistry.AI and other top dentists are enhancing the AI-based caries detection software.[19]

Artificial intelligence allows Dentistry.AI to rapidly discover caries on dental x-rays. Furthermore, the AI-based technology seamlessly integrates with different X-ray sensors and detects caries within seconds.

Evidentiae

Evidentiae is creative and innovative cloud-based dental software with a streamlined virtual workflow. Its algorithm is created to pull information from dental and medical histories and charted exam results to generate a comprehensive overview of patients' dental health. It builds an in-depth diagnostics opinion for functional decision-making, biochemical parameters, dentofacial alterations, and, of course, periodical concerns.

Furthermore, Evidentiae is created to give dentists the most comprehensive documentation currently available, with the ability to use the provided information in the event of a presentation.

Advantages of AI in Dentistry

a) AI algorithms can perform various dental tasks in less time as compared to conventional methods.

b) It helps in achieving a greater degree of accuracy and precision by reducing human errors.

c) AI can store and keep patient data regarding dental problems in a single place and enables the dentist to make a more accurate diagnosis.

d) Prediction of various dental problems can be made by using databases containing millions of symptoms and diagnoses of particular dental diseases.

Limitations of AI in Dentistry

a) Its setup requires immense expenses due to the use of new and complex machines.

b) Properly trained professionals are required.

c) Most of the time, the outcomes of AI do not apply to real-world dentistry.

In conclusion, the world will experience the birth of AI-based technologies in the healthcare industry, including dentistry. These technologies will eliminate virtually all the repetitive manual and digital tasks. AI models can be applied for quick diagnosis and treatment of complex dental problems. AI has a bright future in both maxillofacial radiology and general dentistry. Very soon, we will see AI being applied in most tasks in endodontics, orthodontics, and restorative dentistry.

References/Further Reading

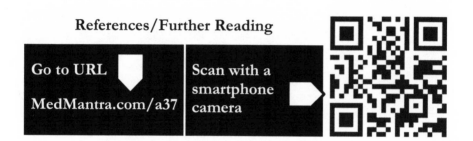

Go to URL

MedMantra.com/a37

Scan with a smartphone camera

CHAPTER TWENTY
ORTHOPEDICS

Machine learning intended to derive information about treatment patterns and diagnoses has already been utilized in more massive digital databases of Electronic Health Records (EHR) in the UK and has enhanced the data-based prediction of drug effects and interactions, the discovery of comorbidity clusters in autism spectrum disorders, and the identification of type 2 diabetes subgroups.

The United States is not left behind either, as the IBM Watson Health cognitive computing system (IBM Corp., Armonk, New York) used machine learning (ML) approaches to develop a decision support system for doctors treating cancer patients in order to improve diagnostic accuracy and reduce costs using large volumes of patient cases and more than one million scholarly articles.

Furthermore, within musculoskeletal medicine, active shape modeling and machine learning are influential in the comprehension of orthopedics, biomechanics, robotic surgery, bone tumor resection, and prediction of the progression of osteoarthritis based on anatomical shape assessment.

Over the years, we have come to realize that machine learning and deep learning are changing the present medical, and especially the musculoskeletal, landscape. Moreover, through the power of search engines, voice recognition, spam filters, and, of course, autonomous driving vehicles all rely on machine learning technologies and are presently part of our lives, no matter which industry sector we belong to. Furthermore, medicine seems particularly receptive to machine learning solutions, and it has been the center of interest in developing technological economies like those in Silicon Valley.

Artificial intelligence and orthopedics

According to the Bone & Joint Research, significant improvements have been seen in all phases of the medical imaging pathway, from analysis and interpretation to acquisition and reconstruction.

Segmentation

Segmentation, which is the division of digitized images into homogeneous partitions concerning specific borders of regions of interest, is frequently used in the evaluation of cartilage lesions.

Traditionally performed manually

Conventionally performed manually, it is a time-consuming and difficult task with limited standardization. Fully automated machine learning analysis segmentation of wrist cartilage, hip, and knee MRI images has transformed this process and promises to bring automated segmentation into the mainstream of research and clinical practice.

Complex user-dependent image analysis techniques

User-dependent image analysis techniques—for instance, ultrasound for developmental dysplasia of the hip—are specifically amenable to deep learning techniques. Unskilled users can image people in geographically distant or remote locations; these patients can be accurately diagnosed and then directed to professional care at an earlier stage in the natural history of the disease, possibly transforming outcomes.

Kenneth Urish has been developing an AI that can determine the progression of cartilage loss in osteoarthritis by evaluating MRI images.[1] There is evidence that AI can ease the grading process of lumbar disc pathology with 95.6% accuracy. The use of AI in estimating the age of human bones and finding joint and other bony pathologies has a great degree of precision when combined with the work of a trained radiologist.[2]

MyRecovery

One of the artificial intelligence applications created for orthopedics is *MyRecovery*. It was founded by Axel Sylvan and Tom Harte and is a brilliantly designed app for orthopedic patients. Furthermore, the London-based company's app contains information developed and approved by surgeons who seek to help orthopedic surgery patients feel more informed about their pre- or post-operation care and treatment plan.

The digital health app improves patients' experience by enhancing the flow of information from surgeons to patients. MyRecovery includes tips and advice for patients; it allows them to track their progress on the road to recovery. Moreover, all content is approved by the patient's surgeon, which makes the information specific to the patient instead of depending on a one-solution-fits-all model.

Prediction of the clinical outcome

Patient database, genomic mapping, and radiographic imaging can be utilized by AI to predict the risk and prognosis of the disease outcome. The machine learning abilities of AI can provide personalized patient care by foreseeing the possible complications in various orthopedic surgeries such as lumbar fusion surgery[3], knee valgus[4], etc. Similarly, according to Christopher P. Ames, from the University of California, San Francisco (UCSF), AI can predict the risk of postoperative complications, readmission, benefits, and particular surgical intervention by analyzing the patient's medical and demographic details.[5,6]

Use in the treatment of traumatic injuries

Badylak and colleagues are developing an AI application that can help reduce the duration of wound healing of musculoskeletal tissues by almost half.[5,6] The process involves the use of smart bandages that can analyze the rate of healing of wounds by measuring biomarkers and suggesting an appropriate intervention to hasten the process.

AI-assisted robotic use

The use of robots in orthopedic surgery began in 1992 with the application of ROBODOC in the treatment of total hip replacement.[7] Some recent advancements in the robotic field with the advent of the Mako system have enabled us to efficiently perform complex operations such as arthroplasty of the hip and knee.[8] Most spine surgeries done today implicate the use of Renaissance and Rosa robots, which have the finest precision—far better than that of human hands.[9] AI-based spine surgery has greatly helped surgeons to minimize the damage caused to neurovascular bundles during operative procedures such as placement of screws. In 2019, 5G-enabled remote surgery was performed for the first time by Prof. Wei Tian with a higher degree of safety and efficacy.[6] This clearly shows the universality, acceptance, and promises of the use of AI in orthopedics.

AI in computer-assisted navigation

Robotics have been extensively used in accurately positioning the screws and prosthesis or an implant during orthopedic surgery. An AI-operated device called **Optotrack 3020** can precisely locate the bones using infrared rays, which can prove helpful in any bone surgery or grafting. A similar AI, called **Robodoc**, developed by the Curexo technology, uses the intelligence of AI to drill a canal for prosthesis utilizing CT scan images.[10]

Total hip surgery has shown significantly better outcomes using computer-based technology compared to conservative approaches. The cup placement during the implantation of a prosthesis is reported to be more accurate with the use of AI. AI-based use of modern technology has dramatically improved the process of aligning the prosthesis in the course of total knee replacement. Evidence suggests that there is a 32 percent lower risk of the wrong implantation of screws with the use of AI compared to traditional surgical approaches.[11]

Similarly, AI has reduced the complications of ACL reconstruction.[12] It has also been used to surgically treat fractures and dysplasia of the shoulder joint by making use of the advanced navigation system.

AI-aided radiograph analysis

The AI radiographic analyzer was developed by researchers at the Royal Institute of Technology in Sweden. The use of machine learning has proven advantageous in analyzing radiographic images to diagnose subtle abnormalities, which can be highly useful in an emergency setup.[13]

Multiple pathological images were sent to the computer network. The machine-learning algorithm correctly analyzed thousands of such radiographs and, hence, was primed to diagnose the pathology. The accuracy of fracture diagnosis was 83%, while the accuracy by a human is around 82%. In another group of images, the computer network demonstrated 99% accuracy in determining the body part included in the radiograph. This is almost comparable to the accuracy of a top-rated human-level performance. The future of AI in the field of orthopedics is fascinating, with skyrocketing advancements made every day.

Conclusion

The use of AI has only begun to advance. Although it has revolutionized today's healthcare system, it is still not perfect. The promising boon of AI is accompanied by philosophical, financial, legal, and technical challenges. The use of AI comes with an achingly high financial burden to the patient and the country overall. Expensive healthcare again presents the question of affordability and accessibility. It requires a very high degree of skill to operate AI-powered devices. The cost and time of training are also tremendously increased. While empathy, communication, and emotions are the core human qualities in any field of medicine, the use of AI may hinder a strong doctor-patient relationship.

The recording of a patient database can create the risk of breaching patients' confidentiality. This, again, presents a distinct set of ethical issues to consider. Another philosophical dilemma regards the replacement of human jobs by AI because of the latter's higher efficiency in every human discipline. Also, in the event of medical mishaps arising from the use of the AI device, there are legal implications as to who—i.e., the doctor or the manufacturer—will be responsible for the negligence. These questions should be properly addressed before we move to the real AI age.

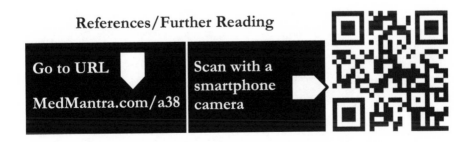

References/Further Reading

Go to URL

MedMantra.com/a38

Scan with a smartphone camera

CHAPTER TWENTY-ONE

OPHTHALMOLOGY

Ophthalmologists are using artificial intelligence, deep learning, and machine learning to verify read images, disease diagnoses, improve surgical results as well as for perfecting IOL calculations, as these modern techniques become more commonplace in the area.

According to Aaron Y. Lee, MD, of UW Medicine, "Most recent breakthroughs have been in the field of deep learning." He further stated that the breakthroughs in computer vision have allowed near-human performance on many tasks in the last 4 or 5 years.[1]

He pointed out that "the Food and Drug Administration (FDA) has recently approved the use of machine learning algorithm for the purpose of automated diabetic retinopathy grading." This is excellent news because it paves the way for AI-based tech to deliver care to a more substantial number of people. Lee believes that the algorithm will play an innovative role in the delivery of healthcare and the way optometrists practice ophthalmology.

Google's Algorithm

The tech-giant Google is not keeping still in the artificial intelligence for improving the practice of ophthalmology. Research teams at Google's AI laboratory successfully trained an algorithm to diagnose a commonly occurring eye disease, as well as an experienced ophthalmologist.[2]

According to Will Knight in "An AI Ophthalmologist Shows How Machine Learning May Transform Medicine," "Google researchers have developed a retinal scanning algorithm to discover out on its own with the much-needed help from humans. It is created to find a common form of blindness; Google's algorithm shows the possibilities for artificial intelligence to change medicine in the near future positively," he said.

Furthermore, Google's new algorithm can scan the retinal images and diagnose and grade diabetic retinopathy, which affects almost a third of diabetes patients, just as a professional ophthalmologist can do. Nonetheless, we can use the machine-learning technique created by Google to tag web images.

In Will Knight's article, he wrote, "Diabetic retinopathy is caused by damage to blood vessels in the eye and results in a steady degeneration of vision. However, if detected early, it can be treated, but the patients may experience no symptoms in the early stage, which makes the screening essential. Diabetic retinopathy is diagnosed in part by an expert who examines the images of the sufferer's retina, captured with a specialized device, for signs of fluid leakage and bleeding".

Artificial Intelligence-based model vs. Traditional model

Lee further stated that the most exciting areas of AI applications in ophthalmology are the areas of personalized medicine and future prognosis. Unlike the traditional statistical models used for risk prediction, AI deep learning models are more flexible and powerful. For instance, deep learning models may have the ability to read a Humphrey visual field and predict how fast they can go blind or understand an Optical Coherence Tomography and predict who will develop wet macular degeneration.

Furthermore, the birth of artificial intelligence has given rise to other possibilities to take place in the healthcare sector, especially in ophthalmology, such as simple deep learning with convolutional neural networks (CNN), automated detectors, disease feature-based versus image-based ("black box") learning, basic machine learning, and advanced machine learning.

References/Further Reading

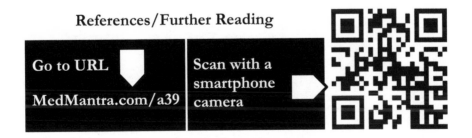

Go to URL

MedMantra.com/a39

Scan with a smartphone camera

"Whenever I hear people saying AI is going to hurt people in the future I think, yeah, technology can generally always be used for good and bad and you need to be careful about how you build it ... if you're arguing against AI then you're arguing against safer cars that aren't going to have accidents, and you're arguing against being able to better diagnose people when they're sick."

- Mark Zuckerberg

SECTION 3

AI IN HEALTH INSURANCE

CHAPTER TWENTY-TWO
AI IN HEALTH INSURANCE

The insurance industry is the central pillar of the economy by virtue of the magnitude of its investment, the scale of premiums plans it collects, and, more importantly, the essential role it plays by covering the personal health and business risks. The majority of the healthcare spending comes from health insurance, with the private healthcare insurance expenses crossing $1.1 billion in 2017, according to Centers for Medicare and Medicaid Services. This corresponds to a 4.2% rise from last year and constitutes around 34% of the total National Health Expenditure.[1]

As the world population is aging, the current health insurance system is being cut off at the knees with the increasing workload and complexity of claims processing. According to OECD predictions, the current insurance system is incapable of hosting future advances and is in dire need of major reforms. With the new diseases being diagnosed and the long-term treatment of chronic diseases, the insurers will need to invest in ways to handle claims more proactively—a process that is mostly manual and takes anywhere from weeks to months.

Artificial intelligence has been adopted by many health insurance companies to take advantage of this revolutionizing technology in claims processing, insurance package selection, improving cost efficiency, minimizing waste of health resources, and detecting fraudulent claims.

Application of AI in health insurance

Artificial intelligence has the potential to revolutionize all the industries on the face of this planet and is thus known as the 'Fourth Industrial Revolution.' The health insurance industry is no different in this regard. The lack of flexibility in the health insurance industry can be eliminated with the use of intelligent algorithms. For example, an AI system can help in coining customized insurance plans for patients suffering from chronic diseases. The extent of potential gains is beyond the horizon.

Artificial intelligence is capable of contributing more to the healthcare and insurance industry. Machine learning algorithms can augment the expertise of case managers in processing claims. This hybrid scheme will increase the efficiency of workers in the screening of claims and will help them make better-informed decisions. Intelligent algorithms continuously evolve with the increasing flow of data—making their own ever-changing rules and revamping the conventional inflexible methods of claims management. A system operating on such algorithms can precisely flag the errors in claims applications while decreasing the human effort in scratching around for possible discrepancies.

Now, we will discuss how machine learning can help fasten claims processing, detect frauds in insurance claims, the role it can play in minimizing the healthcare expense burden, and how it can be of value in predicting investment outcomes.

Revolutionizing claims processing

A glimpse at the process will help understand the complexity of insurance claims processing and the probability of mismanagement. A mid-sized insurer with around 1.5 million customers gets to deal with 0.7 million claims per year in the name of cost refunds. These claims go through a screening process that requires several hundred workers to check if the claim is valid and make interventions where required.

The whole process drains the human resources of a company only to find the majority of claims incorrect. The workers can decide on the basis of available patient history from hospital forms to accept or decline the claim request—an intervention linked to a specific rule book of the company. The correct interventions are important, as the claims audit procedures absorb precious time, manpower, and resources. However, with this current sluggish system, the health insurers can cut the amount to be paid by merely 3%. It's becoming ever challenging to correctly identify fraudulent claims and is costing both health insurers and providers a fortune.

Machine learning algorithms enable prompt and accurate identification of false claims in a really short amount of time, i.e., in a matter of seconds.

The algorithms are trained on already processed claims data of millions of cases. It can efficiently tag only those cases that need human intervention and defer acceptable cases to automatic processing—that, too, at superhuman speed. The system also comments the reason for rejecting the claim, resulting in a quicker, simpler claims management process.

This way, the auditor can focus on cases that are unusual from 'correct' claims determined by AI. This self-learning system only gets better and better as it learns the results of human intervention in cases it was unable to resolve.

On the client's end, this system requires the least amount of effort to submit claim forms. They simply need to take photos of their hospital bill and submit it from the smartphone app and, within few seconds, receive the transaction slip for the amount credited to their account—simple and insanely fast!

Detect fraudulent claims

Fraud detection in hospital claims can also be empowered with AI. For example, the general cost of hospital treatment in Germany amounts to around €73 billion, which accounts for 30-40 percent of the expenses in insurers' budget. However, the ratio of false claims received is as high as 10%. Identifying these false claims with certainty would benefit both health insurers and providers—a win-win deal.

A software company based in New Jersey is using machine learning algorithms to detect and notify insurers of fraud on its custom insurance platform. The name of the company is 'Azati' and was founded in 2001. The company's AI system is trained on huge data of previously processed claims. Fraudulent claims can be identified by detecting connections between data submitted to the platform and revealed to the health insurance company through digital notifications. If the system detects a potential fraudulent case when parsing new applications, it notifies professionals at the insurance company so that an investigation and possible intervention can be done. The software platform also provides details for flagged claims, describing the points used in making that determination. Azati claims that it has helped an unnamed company detect fraudulent claims with three times more accuracy than before—owing to its AI algorithms, and the amount of precious human time saved is another pearl of it.

Cut the health costs

According to OECD, an estimated 20% of healthcare spending is wasted globally.[2] The Institute of Medicine (IOM) reckons this figure to be around 30%. In light of both estimates, the top 15 healthcare budget countries waste an average of 1,100 to 1,700 USD per person in a year, whereas the bottom 50 countries spend around 120 USD per person in a year. In other words, the average per-person waste of money in the top 15 countries is 10 to 15 times more than the average amount spent on healthcare by the bottom 50 countries. Digging deeper into statistics showed that the factors causing this waste include over-treatment, failure of healthcare delivery, and inappropriate care delivery, which are preventable system inefficiencies.

The human experts working in the health insurance industry are prone to make mistakes, not due to lack of expertise but because human nature is fallible. This preventable human error is a huge burden on the insurance system. AI can change the fundamental way a health insurance system works by suggesting accurate diagnoses and predicting the cost of treatments across different hospitals in a state.

Temple University Health System (TUHS), based in Pennsylvania, has benefitted from AI implementation in this regard. Its employees working on the TUHS health plan were infrequently scheduling for medical appointments that increase the insurance expenses. This was estimated to be causing four percent revenue loss per year.

After working in collaboration with Accolade, an AI-powered platform, TUHS was able to dramatically reduce its healthcare costs. The company official said that they achieved around 50 percent more employee engagement and saved more than two million dollars in one year after using AI. In the next year, those cost savings in health care claims have more than quadrupled—amounting to 9.8 million dollars.

Personalized packages

In countries with private health insurance, like the USA, certain treatments such as cancer care are so expensive that only the privileged with premium insurance plans can afford it. Whereas in countries with socialized medicine, where everyone has access to basic health care, new medical interventions are hard to roll out on a nationwide scale, as the system cannot afford it, decreasing the overall standard of health.

Helping clients decide the insurance plan according to their health status is an arduous process with current rule books. It is nearly impossible to list all the rules that go into policy-making, and it gets more and more challenging with new diseases being diagnosed and newer treatments coming out all the time. This is further crippled by the U.S. law that only permits consideration of a mere five factors for calculating premiums. These factors include age, tobacco addiction, location, the applicant (individual vs. family), and plan category. Analyzing the needs of the client based on this limited data is a shot in the dark.

The health insurers must be able to assess the risk flawlessly in order to offer the right premium. If they offer low price packages, it can cost them a fortune. But, if they go a little above the expected cost, they might lose that client next year. Owing to this, the value of their investment always remains questionable.

Prognos is an example of a platform for health insurance companies that are using AI algorithms to accurately assess the level of risk involved in a particular case. They run predictive analysis on each of the new clients to determine which of the members will cost them more in the long term and which ones won't, so the insurers can disburse their resources accordingly. They have trained their algorithms on a large dataset comprising clinical diagnostics data, with 20 billion records of 200 million patients. It is capable of early prediction of the incidence of disease, need for treatment, hospital readmission rates, clinical trial opportunity, and level of risk involved by running algorithms on more than 30 diseases. This provided us with insight into already existing data that was unseen to human workers and help tune the premiums in favor of benefitting both parties.

Interactive Bots

Gone are the days when customers needed to visit health insurance offices or the insurers needed to send workers to inquire about insurance policies or sign clients, respectively. The ambiguity of health premiums had the clients confused about what treatments are covered by their insurance plans and what is the status of their claim processing request. Above that, the stubborn insurance industry, with its tedious workers and long queues, made it really hard to inquire and extract information regarding insurance status.

AI-powered bots promise a solution to the above-mentioned drawbacks of red tape in health insurance. Chatbots can play a crucial role in the efforts to scale for client's needs. That's not to say that health insurers plan on having a monopoly on chatbots and other AI-augmented fronts. What is surprising here is that the insurance industry, with long hold perception of being inflexible, is investing a fortune in getting their hands-on AI bots. According to the survey by Global Trends Study, there is an average investment of 124 million USD per company in this technology. That's 54 million USD more than the average investment across all other industries listed in the 2017 survey.[3]

Trying to comprehend the differences between term-life versus whole-life insurance can be confusing if you're unfamiliar with the field. A chatbot can help reduce this confusion or even eliminate it by using natural language processing algorithms, thus reducing confusion jargon and increasing the chances of a customer opting for an insurance plan. Also, chatbots are available all the time every day and are not limited to business hours only. No one knows when a calamity will happen—road traffic accidents and life-threatening events can and do occur at all times of the day, requiring an insurance claim. People often find themselves restrained to call within working hours if they need help in filing a claim. A chatbot is online at all times, even during holidays and at night. Also, its performance remains unparalleled with high call volume, so customers don't have to wait for hours before their request is answered.

According to a McKinsey report[4], "Chatbots will be the key source of communication for the insurance customers by 2030, and the human personnel engaging will drop by more than 70 percent compared to 2018. China is already leading in this technology by using chatbots in its largest insurance company, ZhongAn Tech. Around 97% of the time its customers interact with AI bots when they reach out to check the benefits, subscribe for coverage, or submit a medical claim; the remaining 3% of the requests are directed to human representatives."

The AI-driven chatbots are being used by 68% of the insurers, as pointed by an Accenture survey[5], to reach out to their customers. And there are reports that more than 2 billion USD can be saved by health insurance companies by using this technology for interacting with customers.

Conclusion

Up until now, the health insurance industry was not doing enough to serve the clients because of routine stuff burdening the stakeholders. Machine learning is capable of handling the massive datasets that need to be analyzed and processed to streamline health insurance workflows. Artificial intelligence is tantalizing the insurance industry with its promising potential to revolutionize the way claims management works these days.

It goes without saying that AI technologies will play a major role in healthcare management. But looking at the future, the solutions to the challenges faced by health care may not be as easy as we would like to believe. They will require careful planning and participation of governments, the private sector, and the citizens. In anticipation of these future trends, we can expect to see an increased implementation of AI-augmented projects in the health insurance industry among major stakeholders endeavoring to decrease costs and scale-up performance.

References/Further Reading

Go to URL

MedMantra.com/a21

Scan with a smartphone camera

"Most of human and animal learning is unsupervised learning. If intelligence was a cake, unsupervised learning would be the cake, supervised learning would be the icing on the cake, and reinforcement learning would be the cherry on the cake. We know how to make the icing and the cherry, but we don't know how to make the cake. We need to solve the unsupervised learning problem before we can even think of getting to true AI."

- Yann LeCun

ROLE OF MAJOR CORPORATIONS IN AI IN HEALTHCARE

CHAPTER TWENTY-THREE

IBM WATSON – MAKING INROADS IN THE WORLD OF ARTIFICIAL INTELLIGENCE IN HEALTHCARE

Healthcare is a major area that is targeted by tech firms, as artificial intelligence can play a crucial role in the development of healthcare. Healthcare is understood to be a challenging field, as there are various facets attached to it. The room for personalization is perhaps the biggest challenge in this field. Tech experts believe that healthcare will be revolutionized in the future with the help of AI, as significant inroads have already been made in the field. One of the major obstacles that AI can face in healthcare is the fact that it must understand the challenges that healthcare faces.

When we talk about AI being used to improve the healthcare system, we can't ignore the contribution of IBM Watson. IBM Watson Health's basic purpose is to provide a holistic approach toward solving problems and challenges that are currently faced by healthcare professionals. IBM Watson calls them health heroes and aims to bring about a change in how patients are treated and managed. The 38th J.P. Morgan annual healthcare conference made a lot of headlines, as IBM Watson Health's manager highlighted some of the major areas in which IBM Watson has progressed significantly. This chapter will look at IBM Watson Health's contribution to healthcare and how it plans to completely change the face of the healthcare industry in the future.

Current Achievements and Research

We first need to grasp the reality that many medical professionals are currently using IBM Watson Health. Statistics indicate that nearly 147,000 patients have their healthcare plans managed by IBM Watson.

It is interesting to note that the number of people adopting this technology is increasing by the day. Here are some of the current achievements of IBM Watson Health.[1,2]

- **Faster Access to Knowledge:**

  IBM Watson Health's approach toward diagnosing a disease is quite efficient as it helps a medical doctor identify or diagnose the disease. And we're not talking about a common disease; doctors often get people who have diseases that are not easily identifiable. Diagnosing them can be a tough task requiring a lot of research to reach a conclusion. IBM Watson Health essentially gives your doctor the edge, as he/she will have faster access to knowledge and be able to diagnose a patient in a suitable time frame. Basically, as a doctor, you must vet all the information that gets published in medical forums to look for the right diagnosis. However, with Watson, you won't have to go through the arduous process of reading long research papers, as it conducts all the research.

- **Recommendations for Better Treatments:**

  A doctor's role is to recommend a treatment that would be the best option for the patient. For this, the doctor must spend a significant amount of time and prepare many notes in order to properly look into the patient's health and condition and to provide suitable treatment. **Memorial Sloan Cancer Treatment Center in New York** is currently training IBM Watson to efficiently manage a doctor's time and provide recommendations for a patient's treatment.

  IBM Micromedex Clinical Decision Support Solution (CDSS) can provide efficient delivery of evidence-based specialized care. These CDSS tools can support physicians in making clinical decisions by rapidly mining the major libraries of medical knowledge from around the globe.[1] TidalHealth Peninsula Regional Medical Centre (PRMC), serving nearly 500,000 patients annually, is a great example of using IBM Micromedex Clinical Decision Support Solution. It has decreased clinicians' time spent on clinical searches from 3-4 minutes per clinical search to an average of less than 1 minute per search.

- **IBM Watson Can Help You in Your Home:**

It has never been about the treatment you receive inside a hospital. It's about how a patient acts or follows a doctor's advice after he/she is discharged from the hospital. IBM Watson can help a doctor monitor a patient's progress when the patient has been discharged from the hospital. IBM Watson uses certain wearables that are essentially indicators of whether the patient is on the path of recovery or if potential hurdles are in his way. "HeartBit" is the world's first wearable device aimed for real-time heart monitoring through a wearable ECG device. It immediately alerts customers about warning signs by detecting early signs of atrial fibrillation, arrhythmias, and other potential anomalies.[3,4] HeartBit produces about 10,000 data points per second that are transmitted to the IBM Cloud, processed with IBM Watson's IoT platform, and shared or accessed by customers or their relevant healthcare providers. Through this process, a doctor will get notified if the treatment isn't achieving the desired results. Then the doctor can act accordingly.

- **Use of Health Bots:**

Personal assistants in a healthcare setting are a great achievement for IBM Watson. You can be greeted by a health bot that can answer all sorts of questions for you. A hospital environment is overwhelming for a child, and health bots can make the child feel calm, as they're friendly and can answer whatever question you have in mind.

IBM recently launched "Watson Assistant for Citizens," a new chatbot solution for the healthcare industry, government agencies, and academic organizations to access up-to-date information and guidance recommended by the CDC.[2] Online, by phone, or by text, Watson Assistant for Citizens can answer commonly posed queries such as "What are COVID-19 symptoms?", How should I clean my home properly?" and "How can I protect myself?"

La Trobe University Australia recently deployed Watson Assistant for Citizens to answer commonly asked questions about COVID-19 symptoms, federal and state restrictions, and current university status for all students, faculty, and staff members.[5] At the government level, Andhra Pradesh state in India has deployed the chatbot powered by IBM Watson on the state's health mission portal to answer common queries regarding COVID-19, including central and state government efforts for treatment, prevention, and welfare of the citizens. It is available in the Hindi, Telugu, and English languages.[6]

Currently, IBM Watson Health has a few products that are being offered to healthcare professionals, as IBM Watson certainly believes that these products can make a difference in how patients are treated in a hospital. A patient's overall experience matters for IBM Watson, and the following tools can help a healthcare professional create an optimal environment for patients.

- **IBM Watson Care Manager:**

IBM Watson Care Manager is a tool that can be used to create a personalized plan for optimal treatment. The Care Manager essentially helps one identify the personalized needs of an individual. Then a concise recommendation plan is created that is best suited for the individual. The Care Manager uses multiple care providers and systems to provide a personalized plan—including identifying appropriate treatments and care—for the patient. Watson Care Manager essentially integrates all the facets of a patient's disease while taking into account care management workflows and third-party system integration. Watson Care Manager is helping greatly amid COVID-19. It supports contact tracing with the help of structured interviews to view hotspots, recovery timelines, demographics, and more.[7] Watson Care Manager also provides integrated care management by reviewing an individual's COVID-19 lab results, understanding symptoms, and severity, and supporting clinicians in making clinical decisions about appropriate actions and interventions according to an individual's needs.

Following are the overall features offered in Watson Care Manager:

Health summary

1. Structured programs

2. Third-party system integration

3. Watson Health Cloud

4. Intuitive user interface

5. Summarization of notes

6. Care mentor

7. Interoperability with IBM Watson Health solutions

8. Oversight and management tools

IBM Explorys Platform

The IBM Explorys Platform is a tool that can be used to integrate large amounts of data in a healthcare system. Data sources such as clinical, accounting, billing, communities, and patient-derived are an essential part of an optimal healthcare system. Explorys enables a healthcare system to analyze vital key points such as managing quality of services, risk, cost, and outcomes. Preparing treatment models and obtaining exclusive insights is also a part of Explorys, as it can highlight efficient treatment patterns and how a patient can get a personalized treatment irrespective of the complexity of his condition. As mentioned previously, three major areas that Explorys helps you to analyze are risk, costs, and outcomes, which can help a healthcare system achieve optimal performance. Mercy Healthcare is a premier healthcare service provider in Ohio that uses Explorys to prioritize high-risk and high-cost patients.

During the recent COVID-19 pandemic, the IBM Explorys platform has defined a specific COVID-19 cohort, which includes individuals diagnosed with respiratory problems and other potential COVID-19 symptoms in the past year along with current confirmed COVID-19 diagnosed cases.[8] The database contains real-world, longitudinal EHR data, which is updated every week. These Explorys databases provide a timely analysis to monitor changes or alterations in COVID-19 trends.[9]

Following are some of the related products that Explorys offers:

- **IBM Explorys EPM Inform:** Every time a healthcare professional undertakes an initiative, the EPM monitors the progress and updates regularly if the initiative is on track.

- **IBM Explorys SuperMart:** SuperMart is an ultra-fast search tool that you can use to search billions of patient records and facts. It also supports Business Intelligence tools, which allows a healthcare organization to formulate a cost-efficient strategy. It's a great tool for getting in-depth information.

- **IBM Explorys EPM Registry:** Registry helps to formulate an integrated framework of a healthcare system, as it quickly identifies the target population and views data that can empower decision-making and risk-stratified care management.

- **IBM Explorys EPM Measure:** Measure is an integrated framework for correlating billions of clinical, operational, and financial events into benchmarks and scorecards for comparison. Typically, it can be seen as a tool that compares metrics for providers, groups, and locations.

IBM Watson Care Manager is a tool that can be used to create a personalized plan for optimal treatment. The Care Manager essentially helps one to identify the personalized needs of an individual. Then a concise recommendation plan is given that is best suited for the individual. The ability to carve out personalized routines for patients makes the prospect of IBM Watson a positive one, as it will change the way patients are treated in hospitals.

IBM Explorys Network

Countless strides are being carried out in the world of AI and Healthcare. Explorys gives medical practitioners a chance to help devise new ways of improving healthcare systems. The Explorys Network offers medical experts a place where they can network with each other and strive toward the improvement of healthcare systems. The network actively promotes collaboration between diverse medical fields like biotechnology, pharmaceuticals, and medical device innovators so that extensive research can be accessed and used by people who matter.

The network is essentially a secured one and consists of nearly 100 million patient records that can be accessed for research and plan formulation purposes. Obviously, a healthcare organization might face certain challenges, and this platform provides them with a chance to learn from organizations that have been successful in similar situations. The basic purpose of the Explorys Network is to expand visibility beyond a certain boundary and become limitless. One can do this by gaining access to records of another organization for research purposes, as valuable insights can be deduced from the fact that the other organization is well-versed in its respective field. Collect, link, and combine data to reach an optimal answer that can be implemented.

IBM Explorys EPM: Explore

Explore is a tool offered by IBM Watson that helps a user gain access to billions of data files primarily for treatments, diagnosis, and outcomes. Further, Explore enables a healthcare organization to delve deep into identifying gaps in healthcare management, disease hotspots, and inefficient treatment plans. The tool is used to analyze various facets that can be attached to how a healthcare organization is performing and actively suggests ways to improve.

Future Plans in Healthcare

We have seen that IBM Watson is currently making significant inroads in the world of healthcare by using artificial intelligence, but the company's future plans have the potential to revolutionize the healthcare system. Here are some of those plans for improving healthcare systems:

i. *The Drug Discovery Process:*

Statistics indicate that the pharmaceutical industry, on average, takes ten years to identify a new drug that can treat disease more efficiently. IBM Watson plans to accelerate the process of identifying potential new drugs. Interestingly, IBM Watson has already identified five new proteins that are linked with ALS that haven't been previously linked to ALS. The fact that AI can uncover invisible data gives it the ability to search for new drugs at a much faster rate.

ii. *Care Management:*

Although IBM Watson is already being used in care management in health organizations, the usability will further increase as it provides a great form of assistance to medical staff. It incorporates techniques that assess high-risk patients and can prioritize them. It further improves the care management process by incorporating access to patient records and other organizations.

iii. *Cancer Treatments:*

A medical professional will know that a large amount of time is perhaps wasted on identifying how a cancer patient is to be treated. IBM Watson will be able to identify the treatment plan for doctors in treating cancer. This technology is already in use in nearly 155 hospitals, and IBM plans to expand this to more hospitals in the near future.

iv. *Clinical Trials:*

IBM Watson's AI can be used to identify the right patient for a certain clinical trial. IBM Watson uses CTM (Clinical Trial Matching) to identify patients who are suitable for a clinical trial. The need for manually identifying patients for a trial will be eliminated and, hence, no time will be wasted. Due to the ability of IBM Watson to store billions of patient data, the matchmaking process becomes extremely fast, with chances of a mismatch eliminated.

IBM Watson Health is a leader in, and a testimony to, the significant changes that artificial intelligence is making in the healthcare system. The main aim, however, remains to be accomplished. This primarily involves making the lives of patients and doctors easier and more manageable. Humans obviously have a limit in what they can perform in the medical field, which includes patient management as well as research, but IBM Watson aims to be limitless and to bring in a change to the healthcare system in terms of improving its overall performance.

References/Further Reading

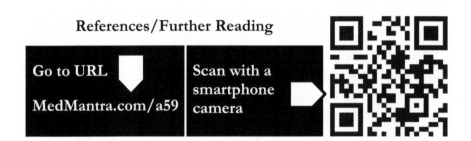

Go to URL

MedMantra.com/a59

Scan with a smartphone camera

CHAPTER TWENTY-FOUR

ROLE OF GOOGLE & DEEPMIND IN ARTIFICIAL INTELLIGENCE IN HEALTHCARE

Artificial intelligence has the potential to change everything we know about healthcare. Perhaps that is why the number of companies using artificial intelligence and deep learning algorithms is steadily increasing. That is also the reason why tech giants like Google are beginning to explore avenues to dive deeper into the medical industry and see what advancements can be made. Since 2014, Google has been branching into various subsidiaries focused on artificial intelligence and healthcare, making an impact on the present and the future.

Google's Present AI Projects

Google's parent company, Alphabet, currently has three main AI projects related to healthcare:

- *DeepMind* – emphasizes AI research in several medical fields;

- *Verily Life Sciences* – analytical tools, research, and partnerships with current healthcare groups under the umbrella of "life sciences";

- *Calico* – focuses on biotechnology and age-related diseases. Not much is presently known about Calico and its projects.

Interestingly, Verily has grouped with the Nikon subsidiary Optos to begin working on detection methods for diabetic retinopathy using AI. Furthermore, Google and pharmaceutical giant Johnson & Johnson recently partnered to create Verb Surgical. The objective of the company is to build a platform for surgeons and physicians that connects robotics, analytics, medical imaging, and more. Although AI is infused into Verily and Calico, DeepMind is the one that holds the most relevance in present artificial intelligence research and development.

About DeepMind

DeepMind was founded in 2010 as a British AI company and was later acquired by Google in 2014. Aside from creating a neural network that allows machines to play video games the same way people do, DeepMind created the "Neural Turing machine," a neural network that can access external memory, thus granting a computer short-term memory like a human brain.

You may have heard about DeepMind's famous success—the AlphaGo program. In 2016, the company became a sensation when AlphaGo defeated a professional Go player twice, becoming part of a documentary film. Another program, AlphaZero, has also beat players in Go, Chess, and Shogi (Japanese game) with only a couple of hours of reinforcement learning. After AlphaGo, AlphaGo Zero, and AlphaZero, in 2019, DeepMind introduced its newest AI agent, called MuZero. MuZero is a significant step forward, and masters Go, Chess, Shogi, and Atari without even being told the rules. The power of DeepMind's artificial intelligence is worthy of respect, which is certainly a reason why Google has been able to weave its presence into the healthcare industry throughout the world.

DeepMind recently launched AlphaFold, which is an AI program developed to predict protein structures.[10] It was designed by using the deep learning system. AlphaFold is currently helping to understand proteins in the SARS-COV-2 viral genome in order to provide useful insights about virus structure and further mutation capacities.

In the UK, DeepMind also developed a diagnostic app called Streams that partnered with the National Health Service (NHS). Oddly, Streams doesn't use AI. Instead, it uses an algorithm designed solely for the detection of acute kidney injury (AKI). Though the NHS ran into issues when giving Google customer data, the app, which was made to aid doctors and nurses in detecting signs of kidney failure in susceptible patients, was welcomed by healthcare professionals at Royal Free Hospital in London. Soon after, DeepMind decided to turn its attention away from Streams for partnerships like the one with Moorfields Eye Hospital. The goal is to train an algorithm to detect signs of major eye-related diseases like glaucoma, diabetic retinopathy, and macular degeneration.

Thousands of scans have been given to the DeepMind AI, and it is now capable of picking out signs of eye disease more efficiently and swiftly than human optometrists and ophthalmologists. The algorithm is also receiving training to use anonymous 3D retinal scans received from Moorfields Eye Hospital to label images for doctors instead of doctors having to labor on their own

Similar partnerships include the University College London Hospital Foundation Trust (UCLH) to allow machine learning algorithms to study MRI and CT scans of patients with head and neck cancer. Moreover, DeepMind and the Cancer Research UK Imperial Centre embarked on a journey to improve breast cancer detection, diagnosis, and treatment in November 2017.

That is just in the UK alone.

Recent Medical Developments with Google in America

While handling the data controversy in the United Kingdom, Google DeepMind has also been working to bring AI advancements to America. Presently, DeepMind and G Suite are trying to solve the ongoing issue of record complications and data breaches. The idea is to create an accessible yet secure method for patient records that adheres to HIPAA regulations. Using cryptography and blockchain technology, DeepMind can encrypt data while lessening the burden of updating and transferring medical data through a network of healthcare professionals.

The incorporation of blockchain into artificial intelligence will hopefully create a more trustworthy network, seeing as how the main issue of data breaches and ethics has already been touched upon with Streams. However, Google, being the internet powerhouse that it is, should have no issue developing an algorithm that does for the healthcare field what others have done for information on the internet and search engine optimization (SEO).

For example, G Suite will handle patient records, meaning that the storage method will be HIPAA-compliant. Because G Suite is "software-as-a-service (SaaS)," physicians with access to G Suite will have the ability to digitally store many medical files, like x-rays, videos, scans, and records.

Google also has its eye on medical video. The Google Cloud Video API Machine Learning system is being geared to sift through media autonomously. Through application to the healthcare field, the AI will be able to rapidly sort through massive amounts of data, thereby finding and potentially preventing sickness, disease, and untimely death. An example of what could one day be possible would be recognizing signs of cancer through ultrasound scan video.

Google Health and the Mayo Clinic recently announced a partnership to develop an AI algorithm to accelerate the process of planning radiotherapy for cancer care. This collaboration will work to build an algorithm for clinicians in differentiating healthy tissues from tumors and planning precise radiotherapy treatment for metastatic tissues.

Conclusion

Google and its subsidiaries in the healthcare realm—mainly DeepMind—are among the many faces of revolution. Though the developments being made by the data and information technology enterprise rely on sensitive topics like consumer data, there is no doubt that machine learning algorithms like those from Google can change healthcare for the better. Already, advantageous steps have been taken. What Google brings humankind in the future will surely have a positive effect on healthcare and the world.

References/Further Reading

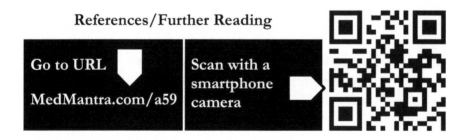

Go to URL

MedMantra.com/a59

Scan with a smartphone camera

CHAPTER TWENTY-FIVE

BAIDU: THE FUTURE OF ARTIFICIAL INTELLIGENCE IN HEALTHCARE?

The future is always near and always full of possibilities. Yet, as many invest in technologies like Amazon Alexa and self-driving cars, some brands are using AI for more unique applications. Baidu, the Chinese Google, was once a dark horse in the technology race but has recently come to the forefront of AI research, alongside enterprises like Alibaba and Tencent. With the bounds in AI research that have already been accomplished, it is safe to say that Baidu could be the future of artificial intelligence.

Software Launches

In 2017, the CEO of Baidu, Robin Yanhong Li, decided to invest in restructuring and rebranding the company, thus placing resources into AI, big data, mobile, and cloud research. Since then, Baidu has developed the following software and devices by pairing up with AI-first companies:

- *Baidu Brain* – In December 2017, Baidu and Huawei partnered to blend Huawei's AI projects with a suite of AI services called "Baidu Brain." This gives smartphone developers access to tools that promote AI-powered smartphones, such as an AI-powered voice assistant. At the same time, Baidu paired up with Xiaomi, another smartphone company, to collaborate on voice recognition and computer deep learning. As of September 2020, Baidu Brain had been updated to version 6.0. Baidu Brain 6.0 was developed with about 270 core abilities and more than 310,000 models for developers, making it a major driver of intelligent transformation for a broad range of industries.

- *DuerOS* – Also known as a conversation AI system, this is a Baidu-powered voice-activated assistant designed to provide recommendations. Baidu built its own AI mobile app that can be used by millions of Chinese, just like Siri or Google Now. DuerOS saw a redesign once Baidu teamed up with 130 partners to make an update happen. Thus, DuerOS 2.0 was born. Qualcomm also stepped forward to help integrate DuerOS into smartphones and IoT devices on the Snapdragon Mobile Platform. Baidu recently announced an upgrade of DuerOS to version 6.0. DuerOS 6.0 is the largest system of its kind in China, has more than 40,000 developers, and receives more than 5.8 billion monthly voice queries. DuerOS V6.0 has also been deployed through the Xiadou AI voice assistant.

- *Little Fish VS1* – Once DuerOS 2.0 was unleashed, Baidu had the chance to introduce a DuerOS-integrated smart display, known as Little Fish VS1, at CES 2018. The device can recognize and respond to different faces and comes with media playback and video call capabilities. Little Fish VS1 also has core Baidu services, such as iQiyi streaming, a cloud photo album, and Baidu Search.

- *Self-Driving Cars* – Out of all the technology giants in China, only Baidu has several patents published for space and autonomous vehicles (15 in the U.S. alone), showing that the company is clearly aiming for the stars. In 2018, Baidu's self-driving software, Apollo, took a car for a spin safely. More than 100 companies, including international enterprises like Ford and Nvidia, decided to invest in Apollo software, and it has gotten the green light for road-testing. Recently, Baidu announced major updates regarding its fully autonomous and remotely driven cars by using the Apollo platform. Baidu also noted that its autonomous vehicles have gone through about 6 million kilometers of open-road testing with zero accidents across 27 cities.[11] In addition, Baidu displayed its fully autonomous robotaxi to carry passengers without the need for a backup driver.

- *LinearDesign*

  Baidu launched the LinearDesign web server in collaboration with the University of Rochester and Oregon State University. LinearDesign algorithms can help giant vaccine companies optimize their vaccine designs based on the most stable secondary structure of the viral mRNA sequence.[12]

AI Cameras to Detect Ocular Fundus Diseases

Baidu and Sun yat-sen University co-developed AI-powered cameras that are deployed in the hospitals of Guangdong province. These cameras can detect three types of ocular fundus diseases, i.e., glaucoma, diabetic retinopathy, and macular degeneration. These AI-powered cameras scan the eyes and develop a report in 10 seconds without the need for an ophthalmologist to be present.

Ongoing Research

At Baidu Research, which has three facilities in Beijing, Silicon Valley, and Seattle, incredible minds have come together to research how AI can be merged with natural language and speech, business intelligence, computer vision, and computational biology and bioinformatics. Although Baidu has pulled back from expanding the AI system known as "Medical Brain," which made waves in the healthcare industry, researchers continue to seek new ways to bring AI into healthcare, finance, and education.

Recent research notes hint at a developing software that provides insight into how people learn a language as well as gives machines the ability to learn. The AI starts blank, but soon, by making use of visual and auditory stimuli, it starts to form an understanding of the language. Once the initial stage is over, the AI unit can start recognizing never-before-seen objects. The teaching environment uses Baidu's open-source XWorld and PaddlePaddle, a deep learning platform.

Baidu is in negotiations with giant investors to raise up to $2 billion in the next three years to support a biotech startup. The Baidu-supported biotech startup will use Baidu's powerful AI technology to perform complex computing for drug discovery and the wide diagnosis of diseases.

With such advancements in technology, there is no clear winner in the race just yet. However, Baidu is proving that with a little reshuffling of one's priorities and partnering up with various international teams, AI can be integrated into everything from classrooms to medical exams, cars to assistant robots. Where will Baidu's vision take us next?

References/Further Reading

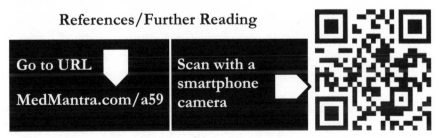

Go to URL

MedMantra.com/a59

Scan with a smartphone camera

CHAPTER TWENTY-SIX
FACEBOOK & ARTIFICIAL INTELLIGENCE IN HEALTHCARE

Facebook has been showing a lot of enthusiasm in redefining the future of healthcare. Through suicide prevention models, Facebook is now showcasing the role of AI in healthcare. It is using AI for the early prediction of suicidal thoughts in users. The main purpose of its AI development program is to learn consumer behavior. The Facebook AI team has conducted several experiments involving hundreds of people. It has advanced its AI activities and is now using AI to prevent suicide. It is making use of various advanced technologies like language processing and speech recognition. It is using user reports as well as human facilitators. When the posts go live, the AI-based software scans them. All signs of distress can be noticed and brought to the attention of the response teams. In this way, Facebook is using AI to rescue humans by combing through video or text data. Facebook has made the reporting options of the site visible to users and can now give information to the concerned authorities faster than in the past.

AI for Fighting the Suicide Epidemic

Every day, no fewer than 20 veterans commit suicide. The same Facebook technology mentioned above is being used to fight this national epidemic in the form of the Durkheim Project. Veterans allow the program to access and analyze their mobile content. If their language indicates a suicidal thought or tendency, the AI software predicts the same. Medical professionals, as well as social workers, are alerted immediately so that they can provide help to the veterans and avert the suicide attempt. The success rate of the initial tests surpassed the rates of the latest methods. Suicidal intent was detected with 65% accuracy, and the software has become a powerful tool for medical professionals to identify people who have potential suicidal tendencies. The government and veterans all over the U.S. strongly supported the project launched by Facebook, whose AI teams are working hard to ensure that all veterans in the U.S. get the benefit of this innovative software.

Saving People from Drug Addiction

Another outcome of this program was the use of AI to detect drug addiction from the data collected using smartphones. Various organizations fighting drug addiction are using AI on mobile platforms. Many new apps are now available to detect drug addiction. These apps collect data regarding screen engagement of the user, phone logs, sleep data, texting habits, and location services. Using the data, the apps help the affected people avoid falling prey to the cravings and triggers that may lead to drug relapse. The information gathered from the person regarding drug preferences, history of drug use, and trigger words is combined with the data collected by the app. AI will provide information about the potential risks and will also send a notification to the person's care team.

Saving Thousands of Lives

Facebook succeeded in showing the world how AI can help people by dealing with serious issues like suicide and drug addiction. AI functions just like vaccines and seatbelts and is saving the lives of many people.

References/Further Reading

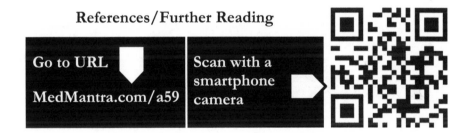

Go to URL

MedMantra.com/a59

Scan with a smartphone camera

CHAPTER TWENTY-SEVEN
MICROSOFT & ARTIFICIAL INTELLIGENCE IN HEALTHCARE

When it comes to well-known names in innovation, Microsoft is an enterprise that comes to mind. Microsoft has done more than develop computers and software that is widely favored throughout the globe. As one of the major players in technological advancements, Microsoft is now joining in on the emergence of a new trend—the evolution of healthcare as we know it. With artificial intelligence and cloud-based data, Microsoft is seeking to transform the health sector.

According to Microsoft, the medical research being done focuses on creating precision medicine and clinical-grade wearables, crowdsourcing health, and increasing accessibility to medical care through the digital world. Other sections of research include genomics, computational biology, and computational psychology. These are no doubt hot topics when it comes to the blending of AI and healthcare. Having Microsoft targeting the same areas as the competition is bound to accelerate the integration of AI into the public sector, as well as increase the demand for machine learning.

Microsoft stated that the "mission at Microsoft is to empower every person and organization to achieve more, and with that in mind, our ambition is that innovators will be able to use AI and the cloud to unlock biological insight and break data from silos for a truly personal understanding of human health, and in turn, to enable better access to care, lower costs, and improve outcomes".[13]

Judging by the research being done, one can say that Microsoft is staying the course.

Microsoft's AI Initiative

In 2017, Microsoft released Healthcare NexT, a program meant to introduce the world to the benefits of cloud computing and artificial intelligence. Some of the projects that have already started to disseminate into healthcare are the following.

AI Network for Healthcare

What was once known as the Microsoft Intelligent Network for Eyecare has been recently renamed to encompass all facets of healthcare. The main objective is to create an AI-based network for cardiologists. It was founded through a partnership with one of India's largest healthcare systems, Apollo Hospitals.[13]

Project EmpowerMD

True to the mission of Microsoft's AI, Project EmpowerMD was launched to create an AI system that can listen to and learn from human doctors to automate tasks in healthcare. If EmpowerMD is successful, AI will be able to handle simpler tasks while physicians can focus on the primary role of their occupation—caring for others and having more face-to-face time with their patients. The project is based on Microsoft Azure.

Microsoft Healthcare Bot Service

Microsoft Healthcare Bot Service is a solution that uses AI to help the CDC and other organizations respond to common queries, thereby freeing up clinicians, nurses, and other healthcare providers to provide the best care for individuals who need it. Microsoft Healthcare Bot Service is an Azure-based cloud service that helps organizations to develop and deploy an AI-powered bot for their patients or the general public.[14]

One of the largest health systems in the US, "Providence," is using an Azure-powered AI chatbot named "Grace" to answer its patients online. Walgreens, the largest drug store in the U.S., has recently deployed Microsoft's Healthcare Bot to support its customers with common health- and medicine-related queries during the pandemic.

Some interesting features found in the Project EmpowerMD framework include services like Custom Speech Services (CSS) and Language Understanding Intelligent Services (LUIS), which are part of the Intelligent Cloud. The use of such voice recognition and language understanding algorithms will be truly helpful in the future, especially for reaching populations that often forego medical care. Smarter chatbots that can recognize certain vocal cues or receive instructions will allow for quicker online consultations and medical treatment. Plus, CSS and LUIS can both be used for translation services, which is excellent for Doctors Without Borders, for example.[13]

Project InnerEye

Microsoft describes Project InnerEye as a way to develop machine learning for the "automatic delineation of tumors" and other 3D radiological images. The goal of the project is to enable the "extraction of targeted radiomics measurements for quantitative radiology," expedited radiotherapy planning, and "precise surgery planning and navigation".[13]

Project InnerEye uses several algorithms already in operation, such as Deep Decision Forests, seen in Kinect and Hololens technology, and Convolutional Neural Networks (CNN). However, the main point is that InnerEye is meant to aid medical practitioners, helping them adjust their practices to redefine results while increasing the quality of care they can give.

Microsoft Genomics

With the main partner for Microsoft Genomics being St. Jude Children's Research Hospital, the primary goal is to cure various diseases. Made from Microsoft Azure, Genomics research provides medical professionals with a powerful cloud-based genomic processing service. Other projects within Microsoft Genomics include Project Premonition, which involves a partnership with Adaptive Biotechnologies and has the ambitious goal of decrypting the immune system.

HIPAA/HITRUST – Microsoft Azure Security and Compliance Blueprint

With the explosion of electronic data and patient records, it is more important than ever to keep information safe, secure, and accounted for. Furthermore, this vast amount of data contains details about various medical conditions, diseases, and treatments that have gone unnoticed because people simply don't have the time to sift through it all. That is why Microsoft Azure Security and Compliance Blueprint for Health Data & AI is a HIPAA-compliant "end-to-end app" that was made to "help healthcare organizations move to the cloud, with security and compliance at the center." Microsoft Azure Security can be paired with Microsoft 365 Huddle Solution Templates or downloaded separately. Presently, groups like IRIS and KenSci are using the Microsoft Azure Security and Compliance Blueprint.[13]

Microsoft 365 Huddle Solutions

In February 2018, Microsoft released new templates based on the original Office 365 platform that are specific to certain industries. Using Microsoft Teams alongside the templates, healthcare groups can enhance meetings and communication amongst one another by using new SharePoint lists, Power BI tables to create visuals, and a Bot Framework for brainstorming and recording new ideas.

Conclusion

So, what does this mean for healthcare? What does the future, where technology and medical care are interwoven, have in store for Microsoft? Undoubtedly, the advancements that are being made by researchers at Microsoft with mapping DNA, enhancing radiology images, and providing swifter, more accurate care are already influencing healthcare systems throughout the world. With companies like Microsoft combining their efforts to create networks like the earlier version of AI Network for Healthcare, which aids in better eye health screening to combat global blindness, or current projects like InnerEye, healthcare is sure to improve.

Many are saying it, but it is true: The future of healthcare is in the hands of technology companies like Microsoft. Without the innovations that have shaped this world throughout the years, many of the diseases and ailments that are already curable would continue to plague humanity. Therefore, these projects from Microsoft are essential to humankind's future.

References/Further Reading

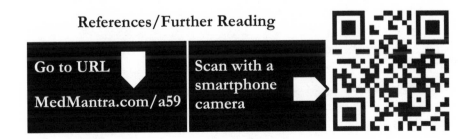

Go to URL

MedMantra.com/a59

Scan with a smartphone camera

CHAPTER TWENTY-EIGHT

AMAZON & ARTIFICIAL INTELLIGENCE IN HEALTHCARE

Structured data is indispensable for training machine learning algorithms. Although electronic health records (EHR) have been here for quite a while, they still contain unstructured text that cannot be used satisfactorily. Plus, hand-written notes, admissions forms, prescriptions, and test reports get buried in hordes of hospital charts, which are impossible to process by bots. Manually sorting these medical records and analyzing them is an incredibly difficult and time-consuming job requiring either medical specialists to understand and input data or developers to write custom codes to extract every chunk of information.

Amazon Comprehend Medical (ACM) is Amazon's answer to this perplexing situation. ACM is a fully managed natural language processing service that can analyze and organize data from unstructured medical notes and prescriptions. It can comprehend medical language, anatomic terms, differential diagnoses, medical test reports, treatment options, medication strength, dosage, and frequency from a variety of non-homogenous documents, making it easy to find important stats and correlate information. The software transcribes doctor's handwritten notes, including medical slang and abbreviations, with astonishingly high accuracy. Amazon says that its algorithm is trained to handle the idiosyncrasies of doctors in history-taking and prescribing treatments.

The use of Amazon Comprehend Medical (ACM) doesn't require any machine learning expertise, and the system can be accessed through an API by an end-user without the need to write complicated rules or train models. A user simply enters the unstructured data into the Comprehend Medical interface, which then analyzes the text and extracts relevant medical data and its interlinked relationships into an easy-to-read format. This can be used to build AI-powered applications for prompt diagnosis and better insights to help doctors make more informed medical decisions. When combined with Amazon Alexa, ACM can also help patients proactively manage their health, including reminders for their medications and booking a visit to a physician right from their home.

Amazon HealthLake

Amazon Web Services (AWS) recently launched Amazon HealthLake, a HIPAA-compliant platform that allows healthcare organizations to smoothly store, analyze, and transform data in the cloud. Amazon HealthLake standardizes unstructured clinical data in a way that unlocks meaningful insights.[15] Healthcare IT giant "Cerner" is using Amazon Web Services as its cloud provider. Cerner's cloud-based platform, named "HealtheDataLab" and hosted on AWS, provides medical data to researchers at Children's Hospital of Orange County for their clinical research and data science work.

Amazon Distance Assistant

Amazon recently deployed a new AI-powered technology, "Distance Assistant," for its employees to maintain social distancing. It works through a 50-inch monitor, a local computing device, depth sensors, and an AI-enabled camera to track the real-time movements of the employees. When employees come less than six feet from one another, highlighted red circles around their feet alert them that they should move to a safe distance apart, based on deep algorithm models.[16]

Privacy has always been a big concern when it comes to cloud computing and massive data flow through machine learning systems. Amazon Comprehend Health is a HIPAA-compliant system that can detect protected health information (PHI) present in the medical data, including name, registration numbers, and family history, and anonymize it to maintain the privacy of individuals.

References/Further Reading

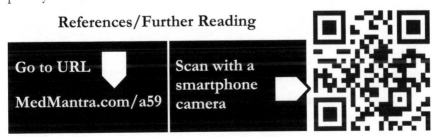

CHAPTER TWENTY-NINE

APPLE & ARTIFICIAL INTELLIGENCE IN HEALTHCARE

AI in medicine will be a $28 billion industry by 2025, and Apple wants a piece of it. The company already has a handsome reputation across the globe and an immense number of users who can help gather health data. This gives Apple a head start on other startup companies and aggregate leverage when collaborating with existing players.

Apple Watch

Along with recording ECG, the flagship feature of the latest iteration of the Apple Watch is the addition of SPO_2 or a blood oxygen sensor, which was added by Apple due to the need during the COVID-19 pandemic. Blood oxygen has been in the spotlight during this pandemic, which has led to a focus on the Apple Watch.

The latest Apple Watch is very popular due to its fitness tracking element along with an app detailing active calories burned. It has a fitness app that detects and shows steps, standing time, exercise running pace, and walking pace as trends. The sleep tracking app in Apple Watch provides a summary of duration of sleep, consistency of sleep, and time in bed. Overall, it may help you improve your routine and overall health.

Apple Health App

The health app comes pre-installed in all iOS devices and is the building block of Apple's AI strategy. The app keeps step count and tracks wellness metrics, including the amount of physical activity, time spent on the phone, calorie intake, and sleep. Also, there are third-party apps to connect with external sensors and trackers to record vitals and other specific biomarkers. For example, there is continuous glucose monitoring through the Dexcom G5 Mobile CGM System.

Apple is now planning to bring EMR data from hospitals into the phone's health record. HealthKit is a software development kit enabled by FHIR that will allow third-party apps to access a health record application programming interface (API). This will enable users to sync their health data with hundreds of hospitals and clinics. For example, a prescription management app, such as **Medisafe,** can access the Health Records feature using API that will allow consumers to import their prescription lists into the portal without manually entering them and also provide relevant information about the possibility of drug interactions.

Carekit

Carekit is a software development kit (SDK) by Apple that enables developers to create apps that can monitor users in real-time using healthcare sensors and tools in iOS devices. **One Drop** is an app built on this framework that keeps track of food intake, medication reminders, and activity. **Glow nature**, **Glow baby**, and **Iodine** are some of the most notable health apps made using the Carekit platform, which keeps users better-informed about their pregnancies, provides information about the natural course of a baby's growth, and helps reduce depression, respectively.

References/Further Reading

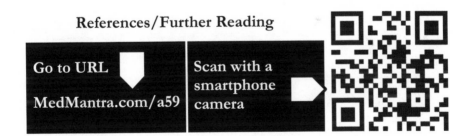

Go to URL
MedMantra.com/a59

Scan with a smartphone camera

CHAPTER THIRTY

NVIDIA & ARTIFICIAL INTELLIGENCE IN HEALTHCARE

Radiology is one of the first medical fields to feel the seismic activity of powerful AI algorithms. The machine learning algorithms can do a superhuman job in recognizing "patterns" in medical images and providing insights to newer dimensions, thanks to blistering-fast GPU technology available today. GPUs are the nucleus of machines being made to run algorithms for medical image processing, and Nvidia is the uncrowned king of this technology.

Powerful GPU Platforms

A sea of health data is available and is being collected by more powerful and affordable genome sequencing gear and smartwatches, intelligent blood pressure monitors, and glucose monitoring devices. Thus, there is a dire need for advanced computing platforms to harvest all this data for use by deep learning systems. **Nvidia DGX systems** are state-of-the-art technological marvels designed to provide the most powerful computing for AI exploration. They are the world's first purpose-built AI supercomputers made to solve the most intricate machine learning challenges.

BGI Group is a genome sequencing center in China that has more than 1PB of data to be analyzed by its machine learning algorithm, XGBoost. By running its algorithms on the Nvidia DGX-1 system, the team shot the analysis speed by 17x and extended the research to millions of targetable peptides for cancer immunotherapy. **United Imaging Intelligence**, a leading AI company, is partnering with Nvidia to deploy its medical imaging software using DGX systems, enabling it to revolutionize imaging workflows, screening radiographs, and treatment solutions.

Open-Source SDK

NVIDIA Clara enables developers to build GPU-accelerated systems and applications to train AI models with an immense number of medical images and automated healthcare workflows. This opens the door to a universal computing platform for developers to build medical imaging applications in sync with Nvidia GPU hardware and bring about a new wave of AI-powered medical instruments for assisting in the early detection and treatment of many ailments. Nvidia Clara promises to bring to the medical imaging field technological advances that have revolutionized other industries, like gaming, self-driving cars, and cloud computing.

Medical equipment augmented with AI-powered supercomputers and intelligent algorithms will be smaller, cheaper, and more efficient, making them more precise and accessible in revolutionizing the medical field.

Health Data Processing

Recently, Nvidia partnered with Scripps to develop deep learning-based algorithms specifically for the early detection and prediction of grave medical events such as atrial fibrillation, which is the predisposing factor of stroke.

To better train their AI models, Scripps is pulling Fitbit wearable data, which is meant to advance precision in the detection of abnormal heartbeats and arrhythmias. Owing to the immense number of users, this will help build a large-scale dataset from more than a million participants.

To give pace to research, Scripps will also provide metadata and key datasets. One such data set contains heart sensor recordings of more than 1000 continuous normal heart rhythms. Another data set provided by Scripps has the entire genomic sequence of people aged above 80 who have never been sick.

References/Further Reading

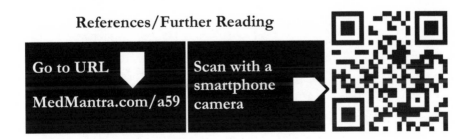

Go to URL
MedMantra.com/a59

Scan with a smartphone camera

CHAPTER THIRTY-ONE

ROLE OF GE IN ARTIFICIAL INTELLIGENCE IN HEALTHCARE

Helping Hospitals Run Smoothly

Hospitals are busy places. Thousands of patients come in daily, depending upon the hospital's capacity. These patients come to different departments. Thus, hospitals generate a lot of data daily. Much of that data is not medical-related and is concerned with the management and administrative point of view—for example, insurance information about the patients, biodata, etc. That data is stored daily but never analyzed due to its sheer size. GE Healthcare thought about this problem and created a system using the techniques of artificial intelligence and deep learning to integrate and analyze this data. The system is called **Edison Applications**. By integrating and analyzing these data from different departments in a hospital, the system can help hospitals run more smoothly. Through this system from GE Healthcare, hospitals can improve their patient interaction by better directing the flow of patients. Analyzing the patient demographics and correlating the data with the frequency of various diseases at different times of the year in different patient groups helps hospitals prepare in advance. In the accident and emergency department, just a few seconds can mean the difference between life and death. This system by GE Healthcare can help save valuable minutes, thus saving lives. The interesting thing about this system by GE Healthcare is that it will do all this behind the scenes. It will be an unsung hero. A hospital will use this system to improve its patient care, and its patients will not even know about it.

Analyzing the Medical Data

Now, that was about the administrative data. However, hospitals generate much more medical data than administrative data. This data comes in the form of patient histories, investigations, patient records, and treatment records. Ninety percent of this data is generated by medical imaging, for example, X-rays, MRI, and CT scans. GE Healthcare has also made a system that can analyze this medical data to help improve the healthcare that patients receive.

X-Ray Scan Revolution

X-ray scanning is the most basic and most commonly used investigation tool in hospitals. It composes around two-thirds of the total medical imaging done. However, nearly 25 percent of the scans fall under the category of "quality too bad to be used." This is a huge number considering the total number of X-ray scans being done. GE Healthcare has created this system to help find the causative factors that make an X-ray of bad quality. It will use artificial intelligence, machine learning, and deep learning systems to find out what makes an X-ray a bad one. It can be many factors: operator-dependent, patient-dependent, or machine-dependent. This system will find the causes and offer suggestions on how to minimize the number of these unusable X-rays.

Tackling COVID-19 with GE AI-Powered Technologies

"Critical Care Suite 2.0," with a new AI algorithm, is helping clinicians evaluate the correct placement of the endotracheal tube when ventilating serious COVID-19 patients. "CT in a Box" is another AI-powered solution to enable fast CT scanning with social distancing measures. It is installed in more than 100 locations throughout the world and greatly helps minimize physical contact with COVID-19 patients. The "Thoracic Care Suite" with AI algorithms can analyze the findings of chest X-rays and highlight abnormalities for radiologists' review, including signs of pneumonia, lung nodules, tuberculosis, and other radiological findings that may be indicative of COVID-19.[17]

References/Further Reading

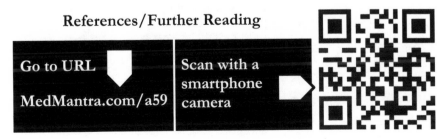

Go to URL
MedMantra.com/a59

Scan with a smartphone camera

CHAPTER THIRTY-TWO

ROLE OF SIEMENS IN ARTIFICIAL INTELLIGENCE IN HEALTHCARE

With the amount of development in the world, access to medical help is becoming universal. More people can afford it. Where it is a marker of a country's development and growth, it also puts more stress on healthcare resources. The medical practice these days has also become very dependent on medical imaging, e.g., X-rays, MRIs, and CT scans. This practice has been adopted to make medical practice and diagnoses more accurate. However, it also means that these medical imaging resources have been stretched very thin.

Proper Utilization of Medical Imaging Resources

Siemens Healthcare has developed a system using artificial intelligence and deep learning to address this issue.

It helps doctors throughout the medical imaging process. Not only does it make the test more accurate, but it also helps in analyzing the reports. It has a three-pronged approach for this purpose.

The Three-Pronged Approach

First, by using infrared and other simple cameras and sensors, this Siemens system helps patients to assume the correct posture and position. Correct positioning is very important for a scan. Nearly one-third of the scans must be done again because of the improper position of the patient. Siemens' system prevents this, decreasing the number of unwanted scans and helping to use the limited resources smartly.

Then, the Siemens system tells the doctor about the vulnerable organs of the patients during the scan. The doctor can adjust the strength of radiation accordingly. It also decreases the number of scan slices if an organ is in a vulnerable position.

Finally, and most importantly, this Siemens system, using the techniques of deep learning, machine learning, and artificial intelligence, helps to analyze the scans and produce an accurate diagnosis. It has a vast database. It has collected this database over many decades from many hospitals. It uses this database to help radiologists accurately analyze scans and provide accurate diagnoses.

Thus, this Siemens system helps to reduce stress on medical imaging resources. It reduces the number of bad-quality, unusable scans and also helps doctors analyze and interpret medical images.

References/Further Reading

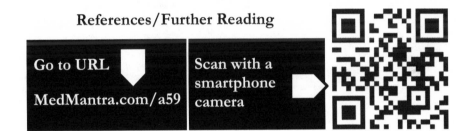

Go to URL

MedMantra.com/a59

Scan with a smartphone camera

CHAPTER THIRTY-THREE
ROLE OF PHILIPS IN ARTIFICIAL INTELLIGENCE IN HEALTHCARE

Philips has many different products that use artificial intelligence systems and deep learning to help the patients as well as the doctors. Let's briefly review the company's products.

Philips Illumeo

This Philips product was developed especially to help radiologists. By using its database and artificial intelligence systems, it helps radiologists better analyze medical images. Using Philips Illumeo for image analysis enables a radiologist to provide better output and feedback reports to physicians whose diagnosis depends upon these reports.

Philips IntelliSpace Portal 12

While Philips Illumeo helps with analyzing images, Philips IntelliSpace Portal 12 has revolutionized the imaging techniques themselves through AVaaS (Advanced Visualization as a Service). Automatic recognition and detection of pulmonary infiltrates in COVID-19 patients is extremely important. The AI-powered quantitative assessment capabilities of IntelliSpace Portal 12 allow radiologists to get useful insights for the identification of COVID-19 pneumonia that is differentiated from other diagnoses.

The latest features in the IntelliSpace Portal 12 include AI algorithms for lung nodule detection, analysis of different cardiac functions, and pulmonary infiltrates associated with COVID-19 patients.

Philips IntelliSpace Portal 12 is changing the imaging techniques in the fields of cardiology, pulmonology, oncology, orthopedics, neurology, and vascular imaging. Their systems are compatible with the machines already being used.

An advanced clinical software package for cardiology is introduced in IntelliSpace Portal 12, which includes MR Cardiac Analysis with CaaS MR

4D flow, to visualize blood flow patterns in the hearts and main arteries of cardiac patients.

Philips Wellcentive

This is an initiative by Philips Healthcare to make quality healthcare available to the masses. Currently, it caters to more than 49 million patients. Patients can get access to healthcare using their phones. It is a health portal. By using the ever-increasing database and sophisticated AI systems, it produces an accurate diagnosis based on the patient's symptoms.

Philips Wellcentive also analyses the population groups for better use of the medical resources in different areas. It also directs its users to the most appropriate healthcare services nearby.

Philips Respironics DreamMapper

Philips Respironics DreamMapper comes with a breathing mask with sensors. This product uses the systems of artificial and deep learning to help patients with sleep apnea get a peaceful night's sleep.

Philips CareSage

Philips CareSage keeps track of the patient's health even after they are discharged from the hospital. Previously, healthcare was limited to the hospital; once the patient left the hospital, no system was in place to continually provide healthcare. Philips CareSage has solved this problem.

References/Further Reading

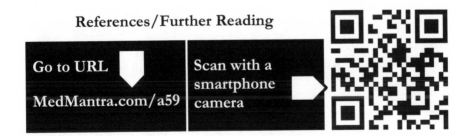

Go to URL
MedMantra.com/a59

Scan with a smartphone camera

"We've been seeing specialized AI in every aspect of our lives, from medicine and transportation to how electricity is distributed, and it promises to create a vastly more productive and efficient economy ... But it also has some downsides that we're gonna have to figure out in terms of not eliminating jobs. It could increase inequality. It could suppress wages."

- Barack Obama

SECTION 5

ROLE OF START-UP COMPANIES IN AI IN HEALTHCARE

CHAPTER THIRTY-FOUR
ROLE OF START-UP COMPANIES IN AI IN HEALTHCARE

Start-ups have long been an influence in the economy by introducing new ideas that either explode with popularity or sink beneath the competition. Now, that power has affixed its gaze to healthcare and seeks to recreate the medical system with artificial intelligence. With some countries struggling to keep up with the demand for thorough and affordable care, as well as low doctor-to-patient ratios, the introduction of these start-ups and their artificial intelligence and machine learning systems may have the answer to all healthcare dilemmas.

For a comprehensive list and description of global healthcare AI start-ups, please visit the "Bonus Content" section at MedMantra.com/aih Here are some of the randomly selected start-ups reshaping healthcare with their artificial intelligence and machine learning technology:

1. AtomWise

AtomWise is a company based in the USA. They use their very powerful AI tools to discover and develop new drugs. Their programs screen for potency, selectivity, and polypharmacology and guard against off-target toxicity with unparalleled speed and efficiency.

The epidemics of the Ebola virus have killed thousands of people worldwide. There are thousands of approved medicines for it. Out of these numerous drugs, AtomWise identified a drug that was not even used as an antiviral drug previously. This drug blocked infectivity across multiple strains of the virus.

2. Medopad

Medopad is a UK-based company that aims to play its role as a bridge between the health care providers and the patients. Its wearables can send data to the health providers so that the patients can get optimum health care with minimum visits to the hospitals. Their strong AI systems also help in diagnosing diseases.

3. VoxelCloud

A Chinese company that is revolutionizing the diagnosis and treatment using AI systems. Their powerful analyzers analyze the medical scans and help in reaching a prompt and reliable diagnosis using AI. The company's current products cover lung cancer, retinal diseases, and coronary heart disease. The company has offices both in China and America.

4. Nuritas

Nuritas, an Ireland-based company, believes in the therapeutic potential of naturally occurring bioactive peptides. They do so by utilizing the knowledge of genomics with the help of artificial intelligence. Their aim is to help different pharmaceutical companies in the development of new drugs and other healthcare items.

5. OWKIN

Owkin is a French company. They have a very comprehensive artificial intelligence program that encompasses many a field. They combine and utilize medical data, the knowledge of genomics, biology, and pathology to reach an accurate diagnosis. They have been making ripples since their inception in France.

6. Insilico Medicine

A Russian company that is dedicated to keeping humans young for a longer time. They use AI systems to research and extend healthy longevity. This company is not limited to developing this youth potion only; they also research and help in the development of new effective drugs by partnering with different pharmaceutical companies.

7. Snap40

A Scotland-based company that makes wearables that take your vitals like blood pressure, temperature, heart rate, respiratory rate, blood saturation, etc. These wearables can not only store them in their data but also send them to your healthcare provider so that they can keep an eye on your health 24/7 with a minimum number of visits.

8. Aidoc

Aidoc is a helping tool for radiologists. Aidoc uses a deep learning algorithm to read medical images. It is very helpful in picking up anomalies from the scans. By helping to read the scans and stratifying the vast data, it helps the radiologists to function more efficiently. Aidoc is an Israeli company.

9. Engine biosciences

A Singapore-based company that is helping pharmaceutical companies to develop new drugs by integrating the knowledge of genomics with medical data using AI. They have introduced a way faster method of drug development, combining high-throughput, massively parallel biological experimentation with artificial intelligence to redesign the way drugs are approached.

10. Fronteo Health

Fronteo health is a Japanese company that utilizes AI to facilitate health care in a system. It helps by applying state-of-the-art word and document embedding techniques and rigorous statistical implementations. They deliver objective, transparent, and reproducible analysis to accommodate healthcare professionals' demands. Some of the fields Fronteo health is playing its part in include diagnostics, pharmaceuticals, personalized health care, and data management.

11. Sword Health

This Portugal-based company was the first to develop an AI-based digital physical therapist allowing the patients for the first time to perform their therapy at home, maximizing engagement and clinical outcomes while ensuring full data accountability. They also make wearables that collect and send the data related to the health of an individual, e.g., Vitals, to the healthcare providers.

12. Lunit

A South Korea-based company that uses deep learning AI technology and the vast pool of medical data to discover, design, and develop powerful data-driven imaging biomarkers. They are especially focused on development in the field of pathology and radiology. Lunit has MFDS approval for AI-powered nodule detection in chest X-Ray scan.

13. Life Whisperer

Life whisperer is an Australian company. It utilizes AI systems to detect the healthiest embryo out of those available. This maximizes the chances of pregnancy following IVF. It takes into account different parameters of embryo health and points out the embryo which is most likely to become a fetus in the mother's uterus.

14. Mediktor

A Spanish company that has put up a very reliable symptoms checker. It uses AI and deep learning to provide an accurate diagnosis. This chatbot has made the availability of health care very easy and accessible. It also connects doctors to patients.

15. Kaia health

A German company which allows your phone to take care of your health. Using AI systems, it is making easy health care available to everyone.

16. Top Data Science

A company from Finland aims to use AI to collect medical data, analyze it, and then point out smart patterns which help the doctors in future diagnoses and treatment of different diseases.

17. Geras Solutions

Dementia is a dreadful disease of old age. Geras Solution aims to start AI systems to help old people with dementia lead a relatively normal life of better quality. It is a virtual assistant helping old people. Geras Health is a Sweden-based company.

18. Triage

Triage is a Canadian company. They have developed this smartphone that can help diagnose skin conditions instantaneously. You just have to take a picture and upload it on the app; the AI system will do the rest.

19. Prognica labs

A UAE-based company that aims to revolutionize the field of oncology using AI. They help early detection of cancer patients with the help of a very advanced AI system that scans and analyses the medical images, giving a very reliable diagnosis. They are also playing their role in helping the pathologists by using AI, machine learning, and cloud computing to revolutionize how histological patterns are read on whole slide images.

20. Qure.ai

This Mumbai-based company was established in 2016. They are using artificial intelligence (AI) and deep learning systems to revolutionize the field of medical imaging. They have developed a large database by analyzing thousands of X-rays, CT scans, and MRIs and integrated their data by using AI and deep learning systems. They proudly present their three products:

i) qXR:

qXR uses AI and deep learning to analyze and find anomalies in X-ray films. qXR can identify and localize 15 common abnormalities in chest radiographs. In its database are a huge number of previous X-ray films and records from the X-ray departments worldwide, so it can give accurate diagnosis even with varying X-ray film quality.

ii) qER:

CT scans are the first investigation to be performed in the emergency room in the case of head trauma. qER detects emergencies like hemorrhage in the brain and skull fractures. qER helps in the triaging and evaluation of patients in the ER, especially in crowded and busy emergency rooms.

iii) qQuant:

qQuant boasts of features, including fully automated detection, quantification, and 3D visualization for CT and MRI scans.

Their aim is to assist the doctors so that they are able to give more attention to the patients.

Conclusion

Artificial intelligence is not only a key to unleashing the potential of healthcare technology; it is the doorway through which we see the future. These startups are just a select few that are revamping the entire medical field with their artificial intelligence and machine learning technology. From streamlining the process of creating and archiving medical records to enhancing medical imaging and detecting diseases, these algorithms and AI systems are backing up the capabilities of professionals throughout the world. As the market continues to shift towards AI-based technology, healthcare is bound to improve—and more startups like these are going to appear.

"By far the greatest danger of Artificial Intelligence is that people conclude too early that they understand it."

- Eliezer Yudkowsky

SECTION 6

CONCLUSION

CHAPTER THIRTY-FIVE
CONCLUSION

The emergence of artificial intelligence in society has gained critical acclaim. While some laud it as an advancement in technology, some schools of thought see it as a necessary evil. But one thing is certain, AI has come to stay, and it can only get better. Some people fear that AI may not be a welcome development because of its immense impact on the job market and humans in general. Most of the time, some people do engage in false controversies about what the introduction of AI may mean to the populace, generating open questions and unlimited controversies about this technology.

So, when are these machines expected to overthrow humans or surpass human-level intelligence? Is it even possible? The problem of ultimate certainty plagues the human race. We have often talked about getting superhuman AI in the 21st century. We often over-hype technology, and AI is in the center of it all.

In the healthcare sector, the use of AI presents many organizations with numerous exciting opportunities. Within a short period of time, healthcare can be drastically improved, that too with saving costs. But there is a need to put autonomous systems in order just in case the deployment of AI may affect the workforce. However, the existence of AI is to be a support system to healthcare givers in various institutions as opposed to the general opinion that believes human employment in the healthcare sector may be threatened by this technology.

Few examples of what AI promises to deliver include scan analysis, sample analysis, taking records of vital signs in patients, and all of which that decide their final treatments by the presiding doctor. The development of new drugs follows some sort of guesswork or deployment of instincts by the scientists who select target molecules from a combination of chemicals. Even though AI is termed the 'experimentalist's helper,' it promises to perform this task with more efficiency and effectiveness.

In understanding diseases, healthcare professionals are skilled at this, but the technology serves as a booster in making better and reliable clinical decisions to fast-track innovations. In short, natural intelligence is supposed to be augmented by AI, and this places it second to human intelligence.

Moving forward...

It has been predicted that AI will hit healthcare in the most shocking way. The predicted steps include:

- Care and management of chronic diseases

- Increasing the availability of health data of patients

- Environmental and socio-economic facets of medicine

- Precision medicine and genetic information integrated with care management

Pharmaceutical companies are also joining the bandwagon of the game of technology, and these people are expected to make the best impact. The development of drugs requires efficiency, which AI is capable of to a great extent.

Nevertheless, the worry that AI may replace healthcare providers is just a product of fear and illusion. The technology promises to be a wingman or a research assistant. After all, what better machine is there than the human brain?

In the not-so-distant future, the expenditure on machine intelligence will be very high, contributing immensely to the business of saving lives. More so, when an error can cost the life of a person, one has to be 100% certain about the procedures. Machines should be given a chance to make this difference.

"People worry that computers will get too smart and take over the world, but the real problem is that they're too stupid and they've already taken over the world."

- Pedro Domingos

SECTION 7
GLOSSARY

Index

Detailed Index

Go to URL

MedMantra.com/a78

Scan with a smartphone camera

Review Request

Reviews are like gold for authors. If you liked this book, please leave me an honest review on any of the following: Amazon, Barnes & Noble, Apple Books, Google Books, Kobo, and Goodreads, or simply send me your personal feedback. I would be so happy.

Review Links

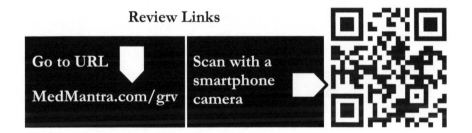

About the Author – Dr. Parag Mahajan, MD

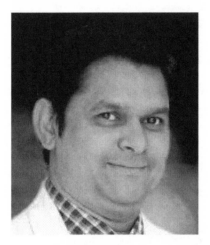

Dr. Parag Mahajan is a radiologist, clinical informatician, teacher, researcher, author, and serial entrepreneur. His current interests include the development of startups in the fields of AI in healthcare, blockchain in healthcare, electronic health records, and medical eLearning systems.

Contact Author

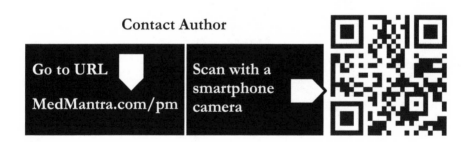

Go to URL
MedMantra.com/pm

Scan with a smartphone camera

Made in the USA
Columbia, SC
27 September 2022

68054719R00164